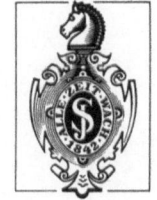

Progress in Pediatric Surgery

Volume 26

Co-founding Editor:
P. P. Rickham

Editors:
T. A. Angerpointner
M. W. L. Gauderer · W. Ch. Hecker
J. Prévot · L. Spitz
U. G. Stauffer · P. Wurnig

Surgery
for Endocrinological Diseases
and Malformations
in Childhood

Volume Editors

M. W. L. Gauderer and T. A. Angerpointner

With 45 Figures
and 33 Tables

Springer-Verlag
Berlin Heidelberg New York
London Paris Tokyo
Hong Kong Barcelona
Budapest

Michael W. L. Gauderer, MD
Rainbow Babies and Childrens Hospital
2074 Abington Road
Cleveland, OH 44106, USA

Priv.-Doz. Dr. Thomas A. Angerpointner
Zenettistraße 48/III, D-8000 Munich 2 (W)
Federal Republic of Germany

Volumes 1–17 of this series were published
by Urban & Schwarzenberg, Baltimore–Munich

Library of Congress Cataloging-in-Publication Data
Surgery for endocrinological diseases and malformations in childhood /
volume editors, M. W. L. Gauderer and T. A. Angerpointner.   p.   cm. —
(Progress in pediatric surgery; v. 26)
Includes bibliographical references. Includes index.
ISBN-13: 978-3-642-88326-2   e-ISBN-13: 978-3-642-88324-8
DOI: 10.1007/978-3-642-88324-8
1. Thyroid gland — Surgery. 2. Endocrine glands — Surgery. 3. Pediatric endocrinology.
I. Gauderer, Michael W. L. II. Angerpointner, Thomas. III. Series.
[DNLM: 1. Abnormalities. 2. Endocrine Diseases — in infancy & childhood. 3. Endocrine Glands
— surgery. WS 330 S961]
RD137.A1P7   vol. 26   [RD599.5.T.46]   617'.98 s — dc20   [617.5'39059]   DNLM/DLC
for Library of Congress   91-4593   CIP

© Springer-Verlag Berlin Heidelberg 1991
Softcover reprint of the hardcover 1st edition 1991
The use of registered names, trademarks, etc. in this publication does not imply, even in the absence of a specific statement, that such names are exempt from the relevant protective laws and
regulations and therefore free for general use.

Product liability: The publisher can give no guarantee for information about drug dosage and
application thereof contained in this book. In every individual case the respective user must check
its accuracy by consulting other pharmaceutical literature.

23/3145-543210   Printed on acid-free paper

Preface

Endocrine conditions requiring surgical intervention in the pediatric age-group are uncommon. When diagnosed, they are the source of great interest and, often, considerable debate. This is understandable, since few centers and even fewer individual surgeons can draw on vast experience of this subject. The great divergence of opinion regarding management is also understandable in that pediatric endocrine lesions often differ considerably from their adult counterparts in histology, natural history and response to treatment. Pediatric endocrine lesions are also, as a rule, less frequently malignant. In addition to the great strides made in surgical and anesthetic technique and operative monitoring, progress in four areas has substantially advanced the management of endocrine disorders in the pediatric age group in the last decade: imaging, pathology, pharmacology and genetics.

The new imaging tools, ultrasonography, computed tomography and magnetic resonance imaging, have added great diagnostic possibilities. More recent developments, such as radionuclide imaging for the adrenal gland and the possibility of using tagged antibodies, promise to expand our imaging horizons even further. In the field of pathology, the development of immunocytochemical markers (e.g., monoclonal antibodies), the refinement in special stains and the continuous perfection of fine needle aspiration biopsies offer great new diagnostic as well as research capabilities. Newer pharmacological agents, such as the alpha and beta blockers, the calcium channel blockers and thyroxine analogs, add a whole new level of safety to the management of the potentially lethal pheochromocytoma. The improved understanding of inheritance patterns, as well as a better definition of the multiple endocrine adenopathies, allows for screening of families and the identification and protection of children at risk.

In the present volume, the reader will find valuable information from experts on some of the more regularly encountered pediatric endocrine lesions that are managed surgically. Although the main purpose of this volume is to update health care professionals dealing with the pediatric age group, it is also intended to stimulate the application of the exciting new technical advances to these endocrine afflictions of children.

MICHAEL W. L. GAUDERER, MD
Cleveland, Ohio, USA

Contents

Sonographic Imaging of the Thyroid in Children.
K. SCHNEIDER. With 19 Figures   1

Surgical Aspects of Diseases of the Thyroid Gland in Childhood.
D. LADURNER and G. RICCABONA   15

Surgery for Benign and Malignant Diseases of the Thyroid Gland
in Childhood.
T. A. ANGERPOINTNER, E. BRITSCH, D. KNORR, and W. Ch. HECKER .   21

Indications, Surgical Treatment and After-Care
in Juvenile Hyperthyroidism.
V. RAUH, H. P. KUJATH, C. REIMERS, and B. HÖCHT   28

Late Results of Thyroid Surgery for Hyperthyroidism
Performed in Childhood.
G. CSÁKY, G. BALÁZS, G. BAKÓ, I. ILYÉS, K. KÁLMÁN, and J. SZABÓ .   31

Late Prognosis of Childhood and Juvenile Thyroid Carcinomas.
G. BALÁZS, G. LUKÁCS, G. CSÁKY, P. BOROS, and I. ILYÉS.
With 2 Figures   41

Parathyroid Surgery in Children.
A. J. ROSS   48

Current Status of Pancreatectomy
for Persistent Idiopathic Neonatal Hypoglycemia
Due to Islet Cell Dysplasia.
R. M. FILLER, M. J. WEINBERG, E. CUTZ, D. E. WESSON,
and R. M. EHRLICH. With 5 Figures   60

Surgery for Nesidioblastosis – Indications, Treatment and Results.
B. WILLBERG and E. MÜLLER   76

Surgical Treatment of Nesidioblastosis in Childhood.
J. DOBROSCHKE, R. LINDER, and A. OTTEN. With 7 Figures   84

Total Pancreatectomy in a Case of Nesidioblastosis
Due to Persisting Hyperinsulinism
Following Subtotal Pancreatectomy.
P. DOHRMANN, W. MENGEL, and J. SPLIETH. With 2 Figures 92

Pancreatic Head Tumor in a Child.
C. DEINDL. With 3 Figures 96

Pheochromocytoma in Childhood.
E. W. FONKALSRUD. With 1 Figure 103

Surgical Treatment of Ovarian Tumors in Childhood.
M. G. SCHWÖBEL and U. G. STAUFFER. With 2 Figures 112

Recent Developments in the Management of Neuroblastoma.
M. L. NIEDER and M. W. L. GAUDERER. With 4 Figures 124

Subject Index 137

Editors

Angerpointner, T. A., Priv.-Doz. Dr.
Zenettistraße 48/III, D-8000 München 2 (W)

Gauderer, Michael, W. L., MD
Rainbow Babies and Childrens Hospital, 2074 Abington Road
Cleveland, OH 44106, USA

Hecker, W. Ch., Prof. Dr.
Kinderchirurgische Klinik im Dr. von Haunerschen Kinderspital
der Universität München, Lindwurmstraße 4
D-8000 München 2 (W)

Prévot, J., Prof.
Clinique Chirurgical Pédiatrique, Hôpital d'Enfants de Nancy
F-54511 Vandœvre Cedex

Rickham, P. P., Prof. Dr.
MD, MS, FRCS, FRCSI, FRACS, DCH, FAAP
Universitätskinderklinik, Chirurgische Abteilung
Steinwiesstraße 75, CH-8032 Zürich

Spitz, L., Prof., PhD, FRCS, Nuffield Professor of Pediatric Surgery
Institute of Child Health, University of London
Hospital for Sick Children, Great Ormond Street, 30 Guilford Street
GB-London WC1N 1EH

Stauffer, U. G., Prof. Dr.
Universitätskinderklinik, Kinderchirurgische Abteilung
Steinwiesstraße 75, CH-8032 Zürich

Wurnig, P., Prof. Dr.
Facharzt für Chirurgie und Kinderchirurgie
Schellinggasse 12, A-1010 Wien

Contributors

You will find the addresses at the beginning of the respective contribution

Angerpointner, T. A.   21
Bakó, G.   31
Balázs, G.   31, 41
Boros, P.   41
Britsch, E.   21
Csáky, G.   31, 41
Cutz, E.   60
Deindl, C.   96
Dobroschke, J.   84
Dohrmann, P.   92
Ehrlich, R. M.   60
Filler, R. M.   60
Fonkalsrud, E. W.   103
Gauderer, M. W. L.   124
Hecker, W. Ch.   21
Höcht, B.   28
Ilyés, I.   31, 41
Kálmán, K.   31
Knorr, D.   21
Kujath, H. P.   28

Ladurner, D.   15
Linder, R.   84
Lukács, G.   41
Mengel, W.   92
Müller, E.   76
Nieder, M. L.   124
Otten, A.   84
Rauh, V.   28
Reimers, C.   28
Riccabona, G.   15
Ross, A. J.   48
Schneider, K.   1
Schwöbel, M. G.   112
Splieth, J.   92
Stauffer, U. G.   112
Szabó, J.   31
Weinberg, M. J.   60
Wesson, D. E.   60
Willberg, B.   76

Sonographic Imaging of the Thyroid in Children

K. Schneider

Summary

High-resolution sonographic imaging of thyroid disorders in paediatrics has become an extremely accurate method and is being more frequently used. The need for scintigraphy has therefore dramatically decreased. The anatomy and sonographic morphology of the thyroid gland (normal findings, variants) in infants and children are presented, as are patterns of thyroid disorders and respective algorithms of diagnostic imaging.

Zusammenfassung

Hochauflösende Ultraschalluntersuchungen bei Schilddrüsenerkrankungen im Kindesalter sind zu einer äußerst genauen Methode geworden, die zunehmend häufiger zum Einsatz kommt. Szintigraphien haben daher dramatisch abgenommen. Die Anatomie und sonographische Morphologie der Schilddrüse (Normalbefunde, Varianten) bei Säuglingen und Kindern werden beschrieben. Die Charakteristika der Schilddrüsenerkrankungen und diesbezügliche Vorgehensweisen bei der diagnostischen Bildgebung werden diskutiert.

Résumé

L'échographie à haute résolution, d'une extrême précision, est employée de plus en plus fréquemment pour obtenir des images des affections thyroidiennes chez les enfants. En conséquence, l'importance de la scintigraphie décline rapidement. L'anatomie et la morphologie échographique de la glande tyhroide (résultats normaux, variantes) chez les nouveaux-nés et les enfants sont décrites. On présente des exemples d'affections thyroidiennes et les algorithmes qui y correspondent en échographie.

Introduction

Diagnostic imaging of the thyroid gland was fundamentally changed by sonography. Now, with the use of high-resolution sonography [7, 16], and especially with computed sonography, many diseases of the thyroid gland can be evaluated in an optimal and otherwise unattainable quality without the hazards of radiation. The capabilities of this new diagnostic method on thyroid imaging and diagnostic workup in children and its perspectives will be discussed.

Röntgenabteilung der Kinderklinik der Universität, Dr. von Haunersches Kinderspital, Lindwurmstraße 4, D-8000 München 2 (W), FRG.

Progress in Pediatric Surgery, Vol. 26
Gauderer and Angerpointner (Eds.)
© Springer-Verlag Berlin Heidelberg 1991

Embryology

The thyroid develops as an outpouching at the base of the tongue (foramen caecum). The anlage descends down to the neck as early as the 8th week of gestation. First functional activity (iodine trapping) can be observed at the 12th week of gestation.

Developmental errors include malposition and abnormal size and shape of the thyroid gland, or a combination of these. Examples are: Lingual and prehyoidal thyroid, thyroglossal cyst, agenesis of one lobe or a superior extension of the isthmus of the gland, the so-called pyramidal lobe.

Anatomy

The thyroid is composed of two lobes which are connected across the midline by the isthmus (Fig. 1). On transverse sections the lobes are pear- or wedge-shaped. The isthmus lies in front of the larynx and upper trachea and is often very thin.

The lobes extend upwards on both sides of the larynx and occasionally down along the trachea to the jugular fossa. On longitudinal sagittal or lateral sections they have an oval disk- or barlike shape (see Fig. 5). The common carotid arteries and internal jugular veins are located at the lateral edges of the two thyroid lobes (see Fig. 1). The left common carotid artery is occasionally found behind the lateral margin of the left lobe. The cervical esophagus is either in the midline behind the trachea or partially to the left. The thyroid is bordered posteriorly in the midline by the cervical spine, the longus colli and scalene muscles, anteriorly by the sternohyoid and sternothyroid, and laterally by the sternocleidomastoid mus-

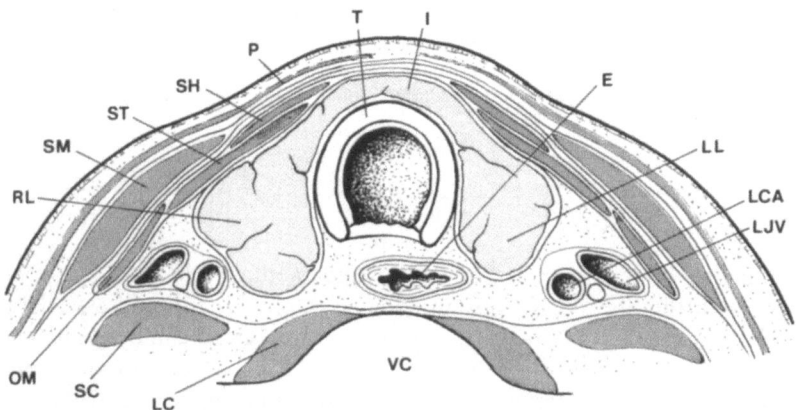

Fig. 1. Anatomy of the neck. Transverse section through the thyroid at the level of the first tracheal ring. *I*, Isthmus; *T*, trachea; *RL*, right lobe; *LL*, left lobe of the thyroid; *E*, esophagus; *LCA*, left carotid artery; *LJV*, left jugular vein; *P*, platysma, *SM*, *SH*, *ST*, *OM*, *SC*, and *LC*, sternocleidomastoid, sternohyoid, sternothyroid, omohyoid, scalene and longus colli muscles; *VC*, vertebral column

cles. The parathyroids are closely situated at the posterior surfaces of the thyroid lobes.

Ultrasound Equipment and Examination Technique

Satisfactory images can be obtained with conventional sonographic equipment using at least a 7.5-MHz linear transducer [7]. However, computed sonography is much better than conventional sonography in delineating morphological details of the glandular tissue. We use a 5.0-MHz linear transducer with a resolution com-

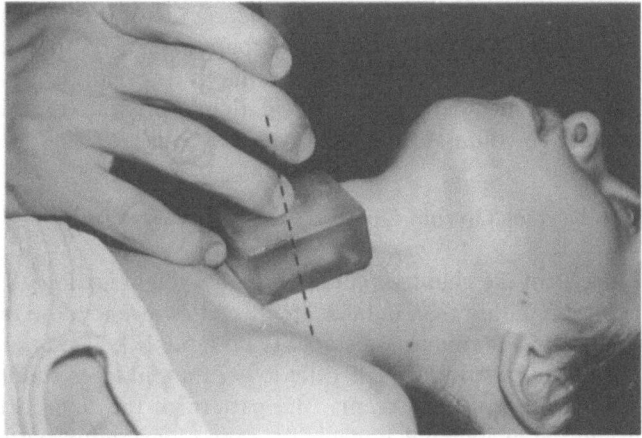

Fig. 2. Imaging of the thyroid. Transverse section at the height of the isthmus. The *dashed line* shows the section level

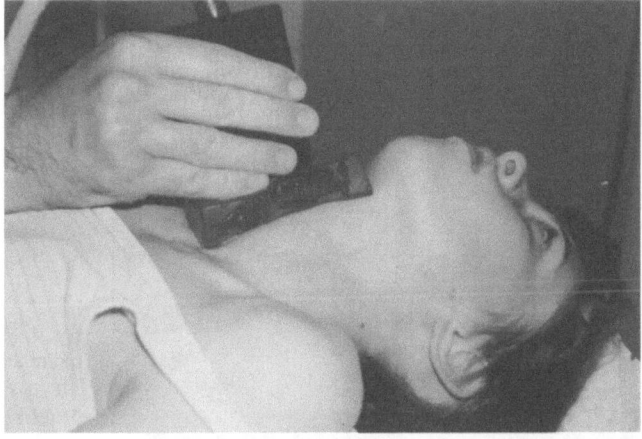

Fig. 3. Imaging of the thyroid. Sagittal longitudinal section through the right lobe

parable to that of a conventional 10-MHz transducer. The use of a water-bath device or a silicone pad is highly recommended [8, 11]. The compound technique is very good but time consuming, and it has been replaced by the real-time technique in nearly all institutions.

The patient is examined in supine position with hyperextended neck (Figs. 2, 3). The neck is imaged on consecutive transverse sections beginning in the jugular fossa and moving upwards to the region of the hyoid bone (Fig. 2). In addition, longitudinal sagittal sections (Fig. 3) through both side lobes of the thyroid from the midline to the lateral part of the neck have to be performed.

With sonography thyroid size and volume can be measured. Measurements of length (L), width (W) and depths (D_1, D_2) of each lobe were done in the horizontal and the sagittal planes (see Fig. 1). The volume of one lobe is equal to L × W × $D_1 + D_2/2 × 0.437$ (cm^3). The correction factor 0.437, instead of 0.523, was found empirically by Brunn et al. on comparative sonographic and volumetric measurements of postmortem thyroid specimens from adults [2]. The volume of the isthmus is not included in these calculations. The total thyroid volume is obtained by adding the volumes of the right and left lobes.

The Normal Thyroid Gland

The size of the gland in relation to body weight is three to four times greater in the newborn period than in later life [8]. After infancy, the ratio of thyroid volume to body surface remains constant at about 5.0 [8]. The parenchymal echogenicity of the newborn's thyroid is a little lower than in later childhood (Fig. 4). In school-age children or adolescents, the pattern of the thyroid tissue changes to a very bright parenchymal echogenicity − the typical adult pattern (Fig. 5).

The thyroid volumes are age dependent (Fig. 6). The daily iodine intake is the single most effective variable related to thyroid growth in children and adults. In countries with high iodine intake, such as Sweden, the thyroid volumes of school children and adults are considerably smaller than in the Federal Republic of Germany [6]. In the FRG the thyroid volumes of children with normal thyroid function are not significantly different from one region to another [6, 8, 9].

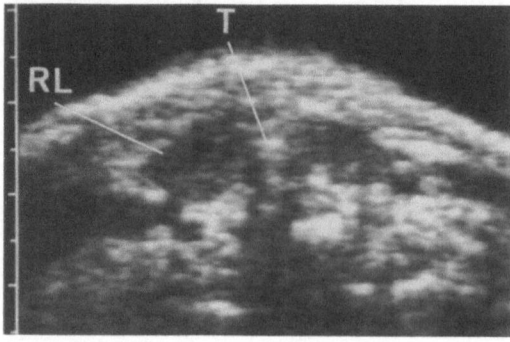

Fig. 4. Normal thyroid in a 4-month-old male infant. Transverse section. The parenchymal echogenicity is lower than in older children. *T,* Trachea; *RL,* right lobe. Compare with Fig. 5

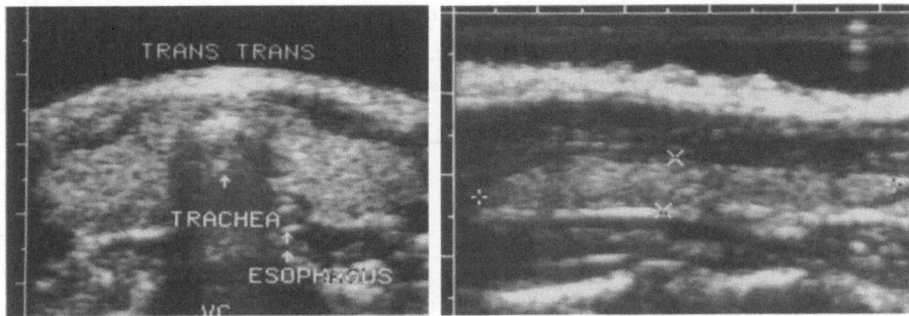

Fig. 5. Normal thyroid in a 14-year-old girl. Transverse *(left)* and longitudinal section *(right)* through the left lobe. *Crosses,* length, depth

Fig. 6. Thyroid volumes (in cm^3) of healthy infants and children in FRG. Normal values for girls and boys [8]

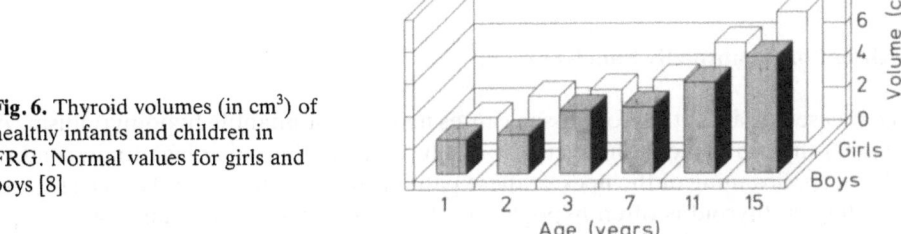

Table 1. Pathological sonographic findings of the thyroid − abnormalities in size

Absent	Agenesis of the thyroid Dystopy (lingual thyroid) Aplasia of one lobe Postoperative status	
Diminished	Hypoplasia of the thyroid	
Enlarged	Whole gland	− Goitre (diffuse, nodular) − Thyroiditis
	One lobe	− Agenesis of one lobe − Cyst, bleeding, adenoma, tumour, abscess

The Abnormal Thyroid Gland

Based on morphology, thyroid pathology can be classified into two main groups by sonography: (a) the size of the thyroid may be abnormal (Table 1); (b) the parenchymal echogenicity can be altered by pathological conditions (Table 2). These changes may affect the whole gland (diffuse pattern) or only a part of it

Table 2. Pathological sonographic findings of the thyroid – abnormalities of parenchymal echogenicity

Parenchymal echogenicity	Distribution of lesions/changes	
	Diffuse	Focal
Diminished	Graves' disease Thyroiditis	Cyst Adenoma Carcinoma Metastasis Focal thyroiditis
Increased	Goitre (iodine deficiency)	Multiple adenomatous changes (bleeding, calcifications, cysts)

(focal pattern). Changes in shape or size and an abnormal echogenic pattern can coexist in the individual case.

Absent or Abnormally Small Thyroid

Decreased or absent thyroid tissue causes neonatal or infantile hypothyroidism. A lingual thyroid gland is the result of a failure of the thyroid anlage to descend to the neck. Scanning of the neck of these patients reveals no thyroid tissue [12]. As the lingual thyroid is often hypoplastic, the ectopic gland itself can easily escape sonographic detection.

Severe hypoplasia of the thyroid was the cause for congenital hypothyroidism in five of nine subjects in a screening program in Italy [3]. Scintigraphy shows no functional thyroid tissue in most of these cases because no endocrine function is detectable [1]. We found one pair of siblings with this rare variant of congenital hypothyroidism (Fig. 7).

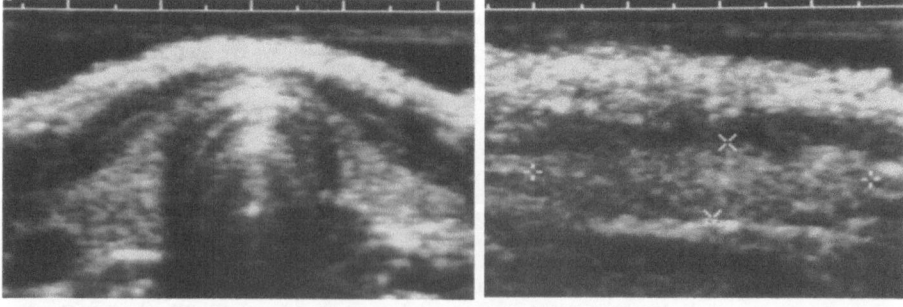

Fig. 7. Hypoplasia of the thyroid in a 24-year-old patient who suffered from hypothyroidism from birth. Very small thyroid with normal shape and slightly increased parenchymal echogenicity. Total volume was 3.1 cm³. Transverse *(left)* and longitudinal section *(right)* through the left lobe

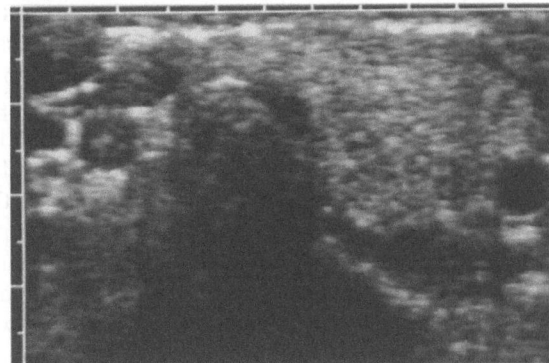

Fig. 8. Agenesis of the right thyroid lobe in a 13-year-old girl. Transverse section shows compensatory hypertrophy of the left lobe

Abnormally Large Thyroid

Visible enlargement of the thyroid is always a pathological finding. However, thyroid enlargement is not always the cause of an enlarged neck [15]. In the newborn, lymphangioma must be differentiated from congenital goitre, which is easily distinguished in most cases by palpation of the neck. However, a specific diagnosis can be made with sonography, because lymphangioma is clearly shown to be a cystic mass, whereas the thyroid appears as an organ with its typical shape and parenchyma. In later infancy and childhood, branchial cysts, lymph nodes or soft-tissue diseases must be considered in the differential diagnosis of a neck mass [15].

When there is agenesis of one lobe of the thyroid (Fig. 8), enlargement of the other lobe is caused by compensatory hypertrophy; in addition, the isthmus is frequently enlarged. The anomaly in these patients may be misinterpreted by scintigraphy as a cold lesion in one lobe [4]. The diagnosis can be easily made by sonography.

Increase of the total thyroid volume is most frequently caused by iodine deficiency. In endemic goitre, there is hypertrophy of the whole gland; the parenchymal echogenicity is at first normal and homogeneous. The thyroid may be-

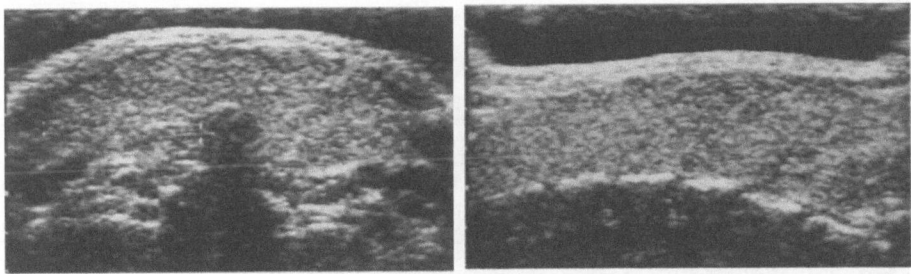

Fig. 9. Endemic goitre caused by iodine deficiency in a 14-year-old girl. Diffusely enlarged thyroid. Transverse *(left)* and longitudinal section *(right)*. *Crosses,* width of the right lobe

come so massive that its lower portions extend into the mediastinum (Fig. 9). These substernal portions extending into the thoracic inlet can be demonstrated in children by sonography, because the ossification of the sternum is not complete until about the age of 12 (Fig. 10). With increasing age, often multinodular adenomatous parenchymal changes accompany simple homogeneous hypertrophy.

Another cause of thyroid enlargement is inflammation. The most common form of thyroiditis in childhood is Hashimoto's thyroiditis, which belongs to the group of autoimmune thyroid diseases [5]. The parenchymal changes during the acute stage are characterized by diffuse decrease of parenchymal echogenicity [1, 11, 13]. The parenchymal pattern is especially inhomogeneous throughout the gland. However, in about 10% of patients with this form of thyroiditis only a general enlargement with no apparent change of echogenicity [11]. In some other cases, focal alteration in echogenicity in a diffusely enlarged gland can be demonstrated (Fig. 11). Associated enlarged cervical lymph nodes are a frequent finding [7]. Histologically, there is a heavy lymphocyte and plasma cell infiltration of the interstitial tissue of the gland. Similar sonographic changes, and sometimes a more marked diffuse hypoechogenicity, are seen in Graves' disease [1, 11]. In some patients acute Hashimoto's thyroiditis may be associated with hyper-

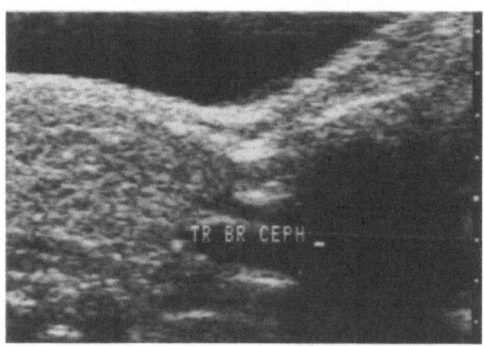

Fig. 10. Same patient as in Fig. 9. Longitudinal section through the jugular fossa. Large substernal portion of the thyroid. *Tr Br Ceph*, Innominate vein

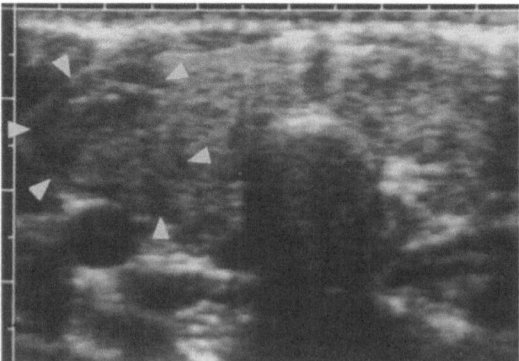

Fig. 11. Focal thyroiditis in a 13-year-old girl with autoimmune disease. Transverse section. The echogenicity of the parenchyma is irregularly decreased *(arrowheads)*, more pronounced in the right than in the left lobe

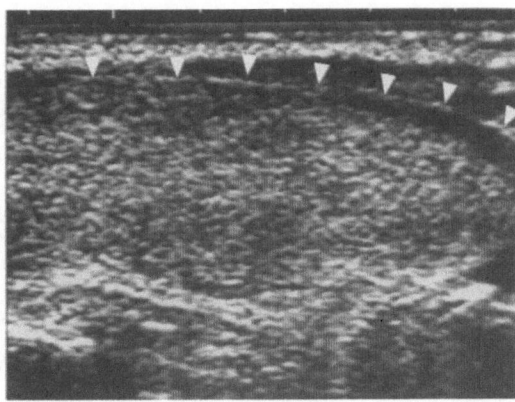

Fig. 12. Graves' disease in a 16-year-old patient. Longitudinal section through the left lobe. The thyroid is diffusely enlarged. The echogenicity is slightly decreased. Halo sign *(arrowheads)*

thyroidism (Fig. 12). However, during the course of the illness the thyroid often decreases in size, and at the same time the parenchymal echogenicity increases in many patients [11, 13]. These sonographic changes are frequently associated with the development of hypothyroidism.

Another form of inflammation is the subacute thyroiditis de Quervain, which in the English-language literature is named 'focal thyroiditis'. The entity is presumably a viral disease of the thyroid which is characterized by a diffuse enlargement of the gland with wandering focal infiltrations of the glandular tissue [11]. Both phenomena (enlargement and focal parenchymal changes) can easily be demonstrated by serial sonography [11]. Characteristic histological signs for this variant of thyroiditis are: granulomas, giant cell reaction, tissue infiltration with lymphocytes and plasma cells.

Solitary and Multiple Thyroid Nodules

Cysts in the thyroid can be very easily diagnosed sonographically (Fig. 13). These cysts are rarely true epithelial cysts. In most cases, these cysts represent degenerative changes in adenomatous nodular goitre. These cysts may contain colloid fluid, yellow fluid (old blood), fresh blood or infected material (suppurative thyroiditis) [11]. Some cysts may have a thickened wall, irregulars contour and/or calcifications within their walls.

The most frequent solitary solid lesion is the echogenic nodule, which is also called adenomatous nodule. More often, however, the whole organ may consist of adenomatous nodules of nearly equal size. In the early stages of nodular development, computed sonography can demonstrate these multinodular changes, even though the glandular tissue appears homogeneous in conventional sonography (Fig. 14). In more advanced cases, the adenomatous alteration of the thyroid is evident. Most of these nodules are echogenic, a few hypoechoic (Fig. 15). In addition small calcifications of some nodules can also be seen.

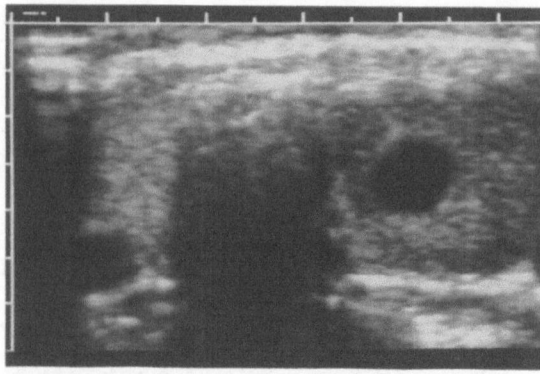

Fig. 13. Solitary small cyst in the left thyroid lobe of a 16-year-old girl. Transverse section

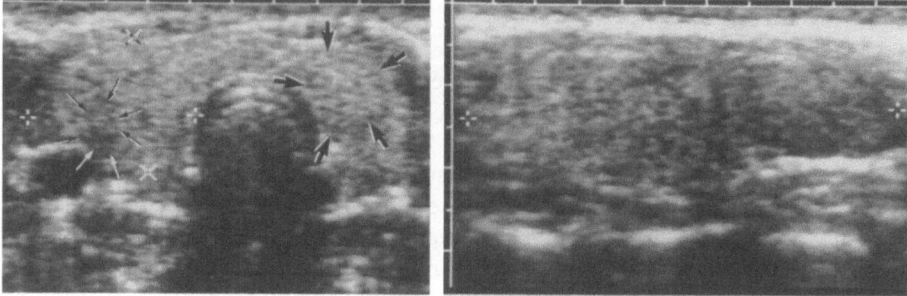

Fig. 14. Goitre with adenomatous changes in a 15-year-old girl. Transverse section shows multiple hyperechogenic nodes *(large arrows)* and very small hypoechoic areas *(small arrows)*. *Crosses,* measurement of width, length and depth of the right lobe

Solitary follicular adenoma must be clearly distinguished from the adenomatous nodules, which are the result of hypertrophy of the glandular tissue. The follicular adenoma may be a functional autonomous nodule (hot lesion in scintigraphy) or the precursor of follicular thyroid carcinoma. Malignant degeneration is unlikely when scintigraphy shows a hot lesion [1, 11]. The follicular adenoma is hypoechoic and in most cases solitary (Fig. 16), whereas adenomatous nodules and follicular carcinoma are occasionally multilocular. The final diagnosis can be made only histologically.

Thyroid carcinoma is the most important nodular lesion in children. Today, early detection of malignant thyroid disease is possible with sonography. Comparable to the detection of follicular adenoma, thyroid malignant tumour is typically a hypoechoic lesion with diffuse borders within a normal-looking thyroid (Fig. 17). Some tumours may be very small; some develop within cysts. In some cases the only positive finding may be enlarged cervical lymph nodes. Computed tomography (CT) is used instead of ultrasound in some medical centres in U.S.A. and Canada [4, 14]. Sonography is the preferable method, because false-negative

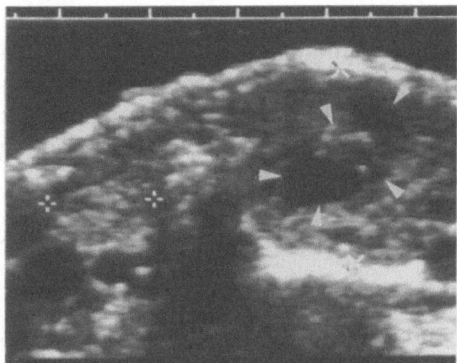

Fig. 15. Goitre with extensive degenerative changes in an 11-year-old boy. Hypoechoic changes located predominantly in the left lobe. Cystic change as a sequela of bleeding into an adenomatous node *(arrowheads)*

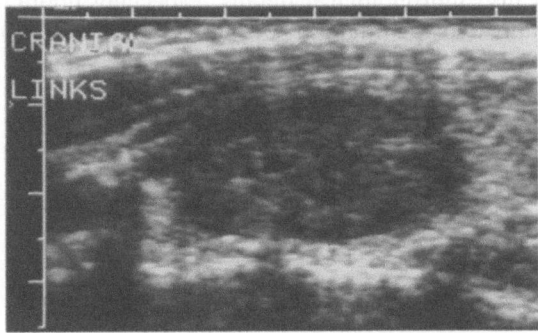

Fig. 16. Follicular adenoma in a 16-year-old girl. Longitudinal section through the right lobe

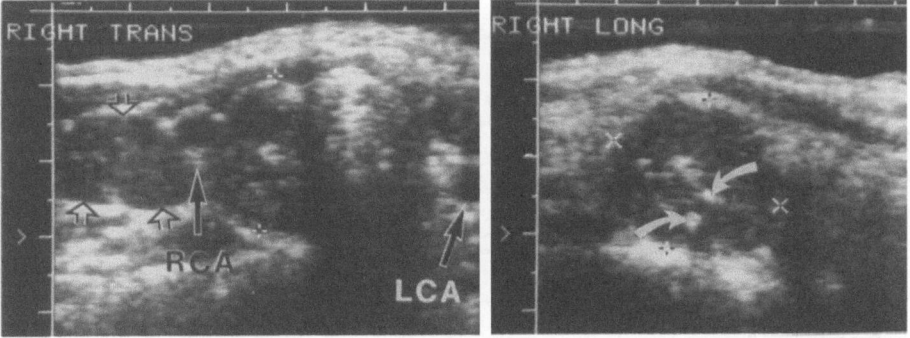

Fig. 17. Recurrent thyroid carcinoma in a 24-year-old woman operated on at the age of 11 years. Lobulated hypoechoic mass in transverse *(left)* and longitudinal *(right)* sections indicated by *crosses*. Enlarged lymph node *(arrowheads)*. Fine calcifications within the tumour *(curved arrows)*. *RCA,* anteriorly displaced right carotid artery; *LCA,* left carotid artery

cases have been reported with CT, the resolution of computed sonography is higher, multiplanar section planes are available, biopsy can be guided in questionable cases and no contrast medium is needed. Recently, high-resolution sonography was proposed as the imaging method of choice for the primary evaluation and even for the follow-up evaluation of patients with thyroid carcinoma [16].

Integrated Imaging of the Thyroid

Three imaging procedures are generally available to evaluate thyroid diseases: scintigraphy, high-resolution sonography and computed tomography (in some medical centres magnetic resonance imaging is also available).

Each method has its specific capabilities. When functional studies are of interest, e.g. with autonomous adenoma, scintigraphy is the method of choice. Because morphological details, especially nodular disease, cannot be fully ascertained by scintigraphy, routine radionuclide studies are no longer justified in thyroid disease in children. The only exception is strong suspicion of an iodine-

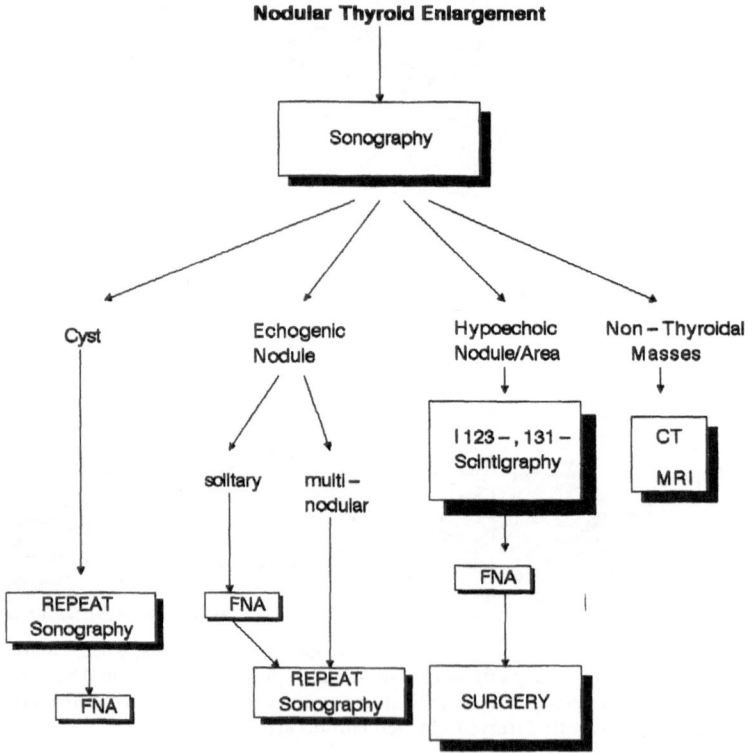

Fig. 18. Algorithm for investigation of nodular thyroid enlargement. *FNA,* Fine-needle aspiration; *CT,* computed tomography; *MRI;* magnetic resonance imaging

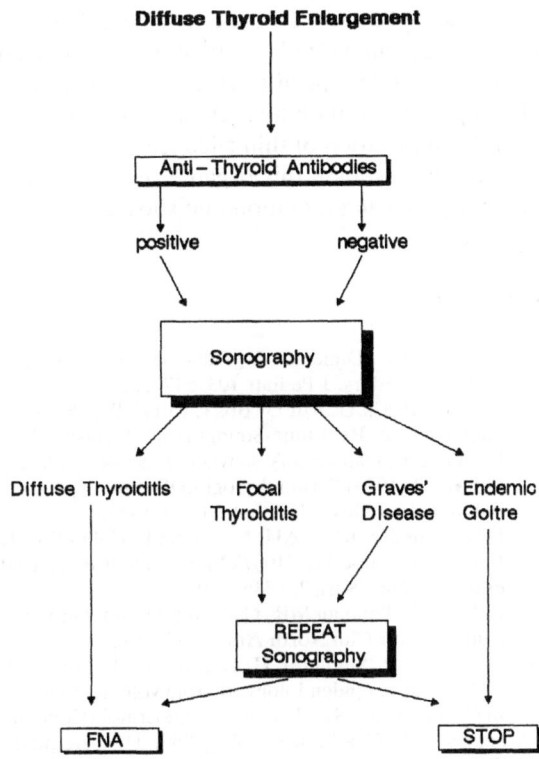

Diffuse Thyroid Enlargement

Anti – Thyroid Antibodies

positive   negative

Sonography

Diffuse Thyroiditis   Focal   Graves'   Endemic
                    Thyroiditis Disease   Goitre

REPEAT
Sonography

FNA   STOP

Fig. 19. Algorithm for investigation of diffuse thyroid enlargement. *FNA,* Fine-needle aspiration

trapping tumour with widespread metastases; then, iodine 131 isotope studies should be performed. Of mere academic interest is the use of radionuclide studies for the evaluation of neonatal hypothyroidism. Scintigraphy is the best method to demonstrate a hypoplastic lingual thyroid [1, 12].

A thyroid nodule should be first imaged with sonography, because the evaluation of morphology of the lesion is critical (Fig. 18). No further imaging is necessary for simple cysts. Multiple echogenic nodules in an otherwise homogeneously enlarged thyroid gland are characteristic for multinodular adenomatous goitre. No further diagnostic workup is indicated.

When a single solid hyperechoic or hypoechoic area or nodule is found sonographically, ^{123}I-scintigraphy and fine-needle aspiration should subsequently be performed. If the aspirate is clearly malignant or not conclusive [17], then surgery is needed. Patients with a high risk for thyroid malignancy should have early surgical evaluation [10]. High-risk disorders are: multiple endocrine neoplasia syndrome, mucosa neuroma syndrome, and prior irradiation of the neck [10].

Fine-needle aspiration is extremely helpful in the diagnosis of focal or atypical forms of thyroiditis [10, 11]. However, in most patients with thyroiditis, thyroid antibodies are positive (Fig. 19); fine-needle aspiration is therefore not needed in the majority of cases.

In our opinion, CT of the thyroid offers no advantage over sonography [14]. Even enhancement with contrast medium does not improve CT differentiation of a solitary nodule. Specific diagnosis is possible only with histology. The resolution of computed tomography is clearly inferior to that of computed sonography, even with the application of thin-slice technique. Imaging of the thyroid with computed tomography exposes this organ − especially radio-sensitive in children − to unnecessary ionizing radiation and should therefore not be used in children.

References

1. Bachrach LK, Daneman D, Daneman A, Martin JD (1983) Use of ultrasound in childhood thyroid disorders. J Pediatr 103:547–552
2. Brunn J, Block U, Ruf G, Bos I, Kunze WP, Scriba PC (1981) Volumetrie der Schilddrüsen-lappen mittels Real-time-Sonographie. Deutsche Med Wochenschr 106:1338–1340
3. Damacco F, Damacco A, Cavallo T, Sansonna S, Bafundi N, Torelli C, Frezza E, Vitale F, Griseta D (1983) Serum thyroglobulin and thyroid ultrasound studies in infants with congenital hypothyroidism. J Pediatr 106:451–453
4. Desjardins JG, Khan AH, Montupet P, Collin P-P, Leboeuf G, Polychronakos C, Simard P, Boisvert J, Dubé L-J (1987) Management of thyroid nodules in children: a 20-year experience. J Pediatr Surg 22:736–739
5. Fisher DA, Pandian MR, Carlton E (1987) Autoimmune thyroid disease. an expanding spectrum. Pediatr Clin North Am 34:907–918
6. Gutekunst R, Smolarek H, Hasenpusch U, Stubbe P, Friedrich H-J, Wood WG, Scriba PC (1986) Goitre epidemiology: thyroid volume, iodine excretion, thyroglobulin and thyrotropin in Germany and Sweden. Acta Endocrinol (Copenh) 112:494–501
7. James EM, Charboneau JW (1985) High-frequency (10 MHz) thyroid ultrasonography. Semin Ultrasound 6:294–298
8. Klingmüller V, Otten A, Egidi R, Seifert-Börner A (1987) Die Schilddrüsensonographie im Kindesalter. Rontgenpraxis 40:260–264
9. Leisner B, Hutter G, Knorr D (1985) Schilddrüsenvolumen euthyreoter Kinder und Jugend-licher. Muench Med Wochenschr 127:909–911
10. Mahoney CP (1987) Differential diagnosis of goiter. Pediatr Clin North Am 34:891–905
11. Maier R (1984) Ultraschalldiagnostik der Schilddrüse. Schattauer, Stuttgart
12. Pöyhönen L, Lenko H-L (1984) Ultrasonography in congenital hypothyreosis. Acta Paediatr Scand 73:523–526
13. Pöyhönen L, Lenko H-L (1986) Ultrasound imaging in diffuse thyroid disorders of children. Acta Paediatr Scand 75:272–278
14. Radecki PD, Arger PH, Arenson RL, et al (1984) Thyroid imaging: comparison of high-resolution real-time ultrasound and computed tomography. Radiology 153:145–148
15. Sherman NH, Rosenberg HK, Heyman S, Templeton J (1985) Ultrasound evaluation of neck masses in children. J Clin Ultrasound Med 4:127–134
16. Simeone JF, Daniels GH, Hall DA, McCarthy K, Kopans DB, Butch RJ, Mueller PR, Stark DD, Ferrucci JT, Wang CA (1987) Sonography in the follow-up of 100 patients with thyroid carcinoma. AJR 148:45–49
17. Van Vliet G, Glinoer D, Verelst J, Spehl M, Gompel G, Delange F (1987) Cold thyroid nodules in childhood: is surgery always necessary? Eur J Pediatr 146:378–382

Surgical Aspects
of Diseases of the Thyroid Gland in Childhood

D. Ladurner[1] and G. Riccabona[2]

Summary

The treatment of juvenile struma is the domain of the pediatrician, and operations are rarely necessary, even in struma-endemic regions. An absolute indication for surgery is diagnosed or suspected struma maligna; relative indications are hyperthyroidism and euthyroid goiter. The operative procedure in benign thyroid diseases is based on the pathogenesis; a tissue-saving technique is mandatory to prevent postoperative hypothyroidism. Therapeutic strategy in malignant diseases, i.e., the radicality of surgical and postoperative management, depends, as in adults, on the prognostic relevance of variable parameters.

Zusammenfassung

Die Therapie der juvenilen Struma ist eine Domäne des Pädiaters, die Operation eine Seltenheit, selbst in Endemiegebieten. Absolute Operationsindikationen bestehen bei Struma maligna und bei Malignitätsverdacht, relative bei Hyperthyreose und bei euthyreotem Kropf. Die operative Taktik bei gutartigen Erkrankungen beruht auf dem Verständnis der Pathogenese, zur Vermeidung postoperativer Hypothyreosen ist besonders parenchymschonendes Vorgehen angezeigt. Die therapeutische Strategie bei bösartigen Erkrankungen, d.h. das Ausmaß der Radikalität der operativen und der postoperativen Behandlung, stützt sich, wie beim Erwachsenen, auf die prognostische Relevanz der vorhandenen Einflußgrößen.

Résumé

Alors que le pédiatre traite très souvent les thyroïdites juvéniles, les interventions chirurgicales restent rares, même dans les régions où cette affection est endémique. L'intervention chirurgicale est indiquée impérativement dans les cas de cancer de la thyroïde et de struma maligna éventuellement dans les cas d'hyperthyroïdie et de goitre euthyroïdique. La technique opératoire dans les cas bénins est guidée par des considérations pathogéniques; elle doit préserver le plus possible les tissus pour éviter une hypothyréose postopératoire. La stratégie thérapeutique, c'est-à-dire le fait de pratiquer une intervention radicale ou non et le traitement postopératoire, dépend, comme chez les patients adultes, de l'importance relative, pour le prognostic, de paramètres variables.

[1]Univ. Doz. Dr. D. Ladurner, II. Universitäts-Klinik für Chirurgie, Anichstraße 35, A-6020 Innsbruck, Austria.
[2]Prof. Dr. G. Riccabona, Universitäts-Klinik für Nuklearmedizin, Anichstraße 35, A-6020 Innsbruck, Austria.

Introduction

Juvenile struma is predominantly a domain of the pediatrician and the pediatric endocrinologist. Table 1 shows the frequency of operations for juvenile struma at the 2nd University Surgical Clinic of Innsbruck from 1972 to 1986. Table 2 demonstrates the incidence of juvenile struma in Austria. Despite the fact that iodized table salt prophylaxis (10 mg potassium iodide per kg sodium chloride), legalized in Austria since 1963, has considerably reduced struma incidence, particularly in children [16], we must continue to consider Austria a struma-endemic country [18]. The situation is quite different in the adjacent South Tirolian area of Sterzing, which is served by our hospital. Legalized iodized table salt prophylaxis does not exist in South Tirol and the incidence of juvenile struma is 48.6% on the average in school children, in some regions even as high as 84% [15].

Although surgery for juvenile struma is seldom necessary, every surgeon should be familiar with the indications and with the principles of operative procedure. The most important relative indications are hyperthyroidism and euthyroid nodular goiter. The most important absolute indication is suspected or confirmed thyroid cancer.

Table 1. Struma surgery in children under 15 years of age[a]: incidence from 1972 to 1986 (2nd University Surgical Clinic of Innsbruck)

Indication for surgery	No. of operations
Euthyroid nodular goiter	3
Graves' disease	3
Thyroid cancer	5
Total	11

[a] Average age: 14 years; sex ratio male : female = 1 : 4.5

Table 2. Struma prevalence among children in Austria[a]

Source	Year	n	Age (years)	Struma Stage I (%)	Stage II (%)
Österr. Statist. Zentralamt	1978/1979				
Austria		51829	Grade	2.1	0.4
Tirol		5041	school level 0.8		0.1
Steiner and Zimmermann [19]	1978	200	1–14	6.5	0.5
Riccabona et al. [16]	1981	–	6–14	12	
R. Ladurner (personal communication)	1986	519	10–14	2.7	0

[a] Iodized table salt prophylaxis legalized since 1963

Hyperthyroidism

Differential diagnostic and surgical considerations are approximately the same as in adults. The kind of hyperthyroidism, the duration and severity of the disease, the size of the goiter, possibly present complications and, above all, the reliability and cooperation of the parents must be taken into account. Hyperthyroid nodular struma is very rare in childhood: there is no such case among our patients. Berchtold [1] reported on five adenomas among 36 operated children with juvenile struma and there was only one case of nodular struma among 75 patients with hyperthyroidism at the Children's Hospital of Philadelphia [21]. On the contrary, immune hyperthyroidism is the form typically seen in childhood. Because of the often transient course of the disease, the mostly minor size of the struma and less psychological stress, thyrostatic therapy is the treatment of choice.

Indications for surgery are lack of cooperation on the part of the parents, recurrent hyperthyroidism following thyrostatic treatment, side effects of thyrostatic drugs and large goiters. Patients with recurrent hyperthyroidism should be operated on as soon as possible, since they are difficult to control conservatively for longer period of time. However, the extent of resection is still a matter of debate. It depends on the recurrence rate of hyperthyroidism and on the rates of hypothyroidism, paralysis of the recurrent nerve and hypoparathyroidism. If one looks, on the one hand, at the problems of treating recurrence and, on the other hand, at the possible spontaneous, unpredictable transition from immune hyperthyroidism to hypothyroidism, subtotal strumectomy must be performed, in our opinion. Moreover, according to our regimen, only those children undergo surgery who are in particular danger of recurrence due to high levels of stimulating immunoglobulins. The rate of postoperative hypothyroidism is high and the condition requires life-long substitution therapy, which in turn makes great demands on the parents' cooperation. For instance, Vaidya et al. [21] reported a hypothyroidism incidence of 37.5% following subtotal strumectomy, Hayles [9], of the Mayo Clinic, an incidence of 38% − in a later series with a more radical surgical procedure even of 50% − and Oberdisse [13] of at least 25%. The postoperative hyperthyroidism rate varies from 2% to 10% depending on the extent of resection [9]. Total thyroidectomy as the most radical form of surgical treatment of hyperthyroidism is contraindicated, particularly in children, because of the implicitly necessary substitution therapy and the higher rates of paralysis of the recurrent nerve and hypoparathyroidism.

Euthyroid Struma

New insights into the pathogenesis of common struma also provide new therapeutic pathways [5]. Identification of immunogenic growth factors in the serum of patients with goiter and the ability of the thyroid follicle cells to proliferate autonomously make it clear why many goiters continue to grow despite thyroxine substitution; why, in struma-endemic countries such as Austria, only about half of the goiters can be explained by iodine deficiency [6]; and why goiters occur even after correction of iodine deficiency, as in Switzerland [4].

With these new insights in mind, the following therapeutic procedure is recommended in cases of juvenile struma: Primary thyroxine substitution; if the goiter diminishes thereafter, the classical TSH-regulated iodine deficiency mechanism must be assumed for the development of goiter. If the struma continues to grow under thyroxine substitution, it can be deduced that thyroid-stimulating immunoglobulins or autonomous processes are responsible for struma growth. In this case, surgical treatment is unavoidable.

Criteria for the extent of resection of juvenile struma are, above all, impending hypothyroidism and struma recurrence. The surgeon should use the following strategy:

1. A particularly parenchyma-saving operation to keep postoperative hypothyroidism, which may have serious consequences in childhood, as low as possible
2. Complete excision of all pathological tissue; otherwise, as pointed out above, a high risk of recurrence must be expected

Table 3. Thyroid carcinoma in children: findings at time of diagnosis

Source	Year	Age (years)	Papillary carcinoma (%)	Male/ female	Affected lymph nodes (%)	Remote meta- stases (%)
Winship and Rosvoll [22]	1960	Under 15	72	1:1.6	76	1
Buckwalter et al. [2]	1981	Under 15	32	1:1.6	47	14
Joppich et al. [10]	1983	–	80	–	44	4
Own cases	1986	Under 15	3/5	1:1.5	3/5	0/5

Table 4. Results of multivariate analysis in papillary thyroid carcinoma

Variable	Parameter	SE (Standard error)	Parameter/ SE (test)	P
Age	0.8329	0.2924	2.8482	0.0044
Local tumor size	1.0822	0.5599	1.9330	0.0532
Regional lymph node invasion	1.3696	0.5966	2.2958	0.0217
Remote metastases	1.7968	0.5890	3.0503	0.0023
Blood vessel avulsions	1.3963	0.5851	2.3864	0.0170
Colloid content	− 1.7908	0.5683	− 3.1509	0.0016

Struma maligna

The incidence of thyroid cancer in childhood is low. Schauer [17] estimates one childhood case among 100 thyroid cancers. Young and Gloeckler-Ries calculate a rate of 1.8 per million white inhabitants in the USA, based on a study by the National Cancer Institute [23]. However, 5 of our 11 patients who underwent struma operations had thyroid cancer.

It must be emphasized in this context that every nodular goiter in children must be carefully investigated. For instance, at the Mayo Clinic, 35% of the operated solitary nodular goiters in children were malignant [9]. Every thyroid nodule that develops under therapy or causes local symptoms and every struma with suspect findings obtained by ultrasound, scintigraphy, or cytology must be clarified surgically. This means, for children as well, a regular operation with complete excision of the nodule, and not just a biopsy.

The predominance of the papillary form of thyroid cancer with primary invasion of the lymph nodes in our patients is in accordance with reports in the literature (Table 3). Lymph node metastases are frequently the first and only symptom of thyroid cancer: Joppich et al. [10] found this to be true in 28% and Harness et al. [7] in 63% of their patients. In the latter series, the average time between first symptoms and final diagnosis was more than 2 years, in single cases even more than 5 years.

In spite of this unfavorable starting position, the prognosis of thyroid carcinoma in children is generally considered promising. Tubiana et al. [20] reported a 20-year-survival rate of 88%, and Buckwalter et al. [2] reported only one death among 68 patients after a follow-up of up to 30 years. Likewise, all our patients are alive and tumor free after follow-ups of up to 14 years. Nevertheless, death due to thyroid cancer can occur as late as decades after surgery [20]. Criteria for the radicality of surgery or of therapeutic strategy in general are the prognostic factors worked out by multivariate studies [3, 12, 20]. Our studies [11] showed the following parameters to be prognostically important for papillary carcinoma, the predominating tumor form in children (Table 4): age, TNM stage, and special histomorphological criteria such as blood vessel avulsions and colloid content. Based on these insights, we are of the opinion that a mere lobectomy on the tumor side is adequate in the rare childhood thyroid carcinoma without remote metastases or unfavorable prognostic factors. If the cervical lymph nodes are affected − the most common finding in children − additional subtotal, contralateral strumectomy with removal of the cervical lymph nodes is the method of choice.

References

1. Berchtold R (1983) Juvenile Struma. In: Steiner H, Galvan G (eds) Die Therapie der Schilddrüsenerkrankungen − Kritisches und Neues. 2. Internationales Schilddrüsensymposium Salzburg, 18−19 Nov 1983
2. Buckwalter JA, Gurll NJ, Thomas CG (1981) Cancer of the thyroid in youth. World J Surg 5:15−25

3. Byar DP, Green SB, Dor P, Williams D, Colon J, van Gilse HA, Mayer M, Sylvester RJ, van Glabbeke M (1979) A prognostic index for thyroid carcinoma. A study of the E.O.R.T.C. thyroid cancer cooperative group. Eur J Cancer 15:1033–1041
4. Eberhard H, Eigenmann F, Schärer K, Bürgi H (1983) Auswirkungen der verbesserten Kropfprophylaxe mit jodiertem Kochsalz auf den Jodstoffwechsel in der Schweiz. Schweiz Med Wochenschr 113:24–27
5. Gerber H, Peter HJ, Ramelli F, Miloni E, König MP, Studer H, Berchtold R, Gemsenjäger E (1983) Autonomie und Heterogenität der Follikel in der euthyreoten und hyperthyreoten menschlichen Knotenstruma: die Lösung alter Rätsel? Schweiz Med Wochenschr 113:1178–1187
6. Grubeck-Loebenstein B, Kletter K, Kiss A, Vierhapper H, Waldhäusl W (1982) Endemische Struma in Österreich. Ist Jodmangel die primäre Kropfursache? Schweiz Med Wochenschr 112:1526–1530
7. Harness JK, Thompson NW, Nishiyama RH (1971) Childhood thyroid carcinoma. Arch Surg 102:278–284
8. Hayles AB, Kennedy RLJ, Woolner LB, Black BM (1956) Nodular lesions of the thyroid gland in children. J Clin Endocrinol Metab 16:1580–1594
9. Hayles AB (1972) Problems of childhood Graves' disease. Mayo Clin Proc 47:850–853
10. Joppich I, Röher HD, Hecker WCh, Knorr D, Daum R (1983) Thyroid carcinoma in childhood. Prog Pediatr Surg 16:23–28
11. Ladurner D, Seeber G, Hofstädter F (1984) Das papilläre Schilddrüsenkarzinom – Prognose und prognostische Faktoren. Langenbecks Arch Chir 363:43–55
12. Ladurner D, Seeber G, Hofstädter F, Zechmann W (1985) Das differenzierte Schilddrüsenkarzinom. Klinik, Prognose, therapeutische Überlegungen. Dtsch Med Wochenschr 110:333–338
13. Oberdisse K (1980) Die Hyperthyreose. In: Oberdisse K, Klein E, Reinwein D (eds) Die Krankheiten der Schilddrüse. 2nd edn. Thieme, Stuttgart, p 189
14. Österreichisches Statistisches Zentralamt (1982) Schilddrüsenvergrößerungen bei Schulkindern 1978/79. In: Österreichisches Bundesinstitut für Gesundheitswesen (ed). Schilddrüse und Vollsalz
15. Platzer S, Riccabona G, Fill H, Ladurner D, Glatzl J, De Sanso G, Brambati-Testori O, Costa A (1975) Notes of endemic goitre and cretinism in the upper Isarco valley. J Nucl Biol Med 19:65–72
16. Riccabona G, Glatzl J, Platzer S, Fill H, Ehlich P, Obendorf L (1981) Gibt es noch eine Kropfendemie bei Österreichs Jugend? Pädiatr Pädol 16:189–194
17. Schauer A (1984) Pathogenese und pathologische Anatomie. In: Becker HD, Heinze HG (eds) Maligne Schilddrüsentumoren. Springer, Berlin Heidelberg New York, p 2
18. Scriba PC, Beckers C, Bürgi H, Escobar Del Rey F, Gembicki M, Koutras DA, Lamberg BA, Langer P, Lazarus JH, Querido A, Thilly C, Vigneri R (1985) Goitre and iodine deficiency in Europe. Report fo the Subcommittee for the Study of Endemic Goitre and Iodine Deficiency of the European Thyroid Association. Lancet 1:1289–1293
19. Steiner H, Zimmermann G (1978) Die Epidemiologie der endemischen Struma unter Jodsalzprophylaxe. Wien Med Wochenschr 128:476–479
20. Tubiana M, Schlumberger M, Rougier Ph, Laplanche A, Benhamou E, Gardet P, Caillou B, Travagli JP, Parmentier C (1985) Long-term results and prognostic factors in patients with differentiated thyroid carcinoma. Cancer 55:794–804
21. Vaidya VA, Bongiovanni AM, Parks JS, Tenore A, Kirkland RT (1974) Twenty-two years' experience in the medical management of juvenile thyrotoxicosis. Pediatrics 54:565–570
22. Winship T, Rosvoll RV (1961) Childhood thyroid carcinoma. Cancer 14:734–743
23. Young JL, Gloeckler Ries L, Silverberg E, Horm JW, Miller RW (1986) Cancer incidence, survival, and mortality for children younger than age 15 years. Cancer 58:598–602

Surgery for Benign and Malignant Diseases of the Thyroid Gland in Childhood

T. A. Angerpointner[1], E. Britsch[1], D. Knorr[2], and W. Ch. Hecker[1]

Summary

From 1970 to 1986, 51 children and adolescents aged 5–18 years were operated on for diseases of the thyroid gland, among them 42 with benign diseases (juvenile goiter 21, adenoma 17, Graves' disease 3, Hashimoto's thyroiditis 1) and nine with malignancies (papillary carcinoma 4, follicular carcinoma 3, medullary carcinoma 1, anaplastic carcinoma 1). In benign entities, females were three times as often affected as males, whereas both sexes were equally affected in malignancies. Positive family histories were found in 23.3% of the children with adenomas and in 71.4% of the children with juvenile goiters. Subtotal strumectomy was carried out in 30 instances and enculeation in 12. Iodized salt and L-thyroxine were given postoperatively as recurrence prophylaxis. Recurrence was seen in two children (4.8%) who had no recurrence prophylaxis.

Symptoms in children with malignancies were palpable cervical lymph nodes and solitary nodes in the thyroid gland. Total thyroidectomy was done in all instances, followed by radio-iodine treatment in eight cases and cobalt 60 irradiation in one case. Two children died, of diffuse metastases and irradiation fibrosis of the lung respectively.

The peculiarities of diseases of the thyroid gland in childhood that require surgery are discussed.

Zusammenfassung

Von 1970 bis 1986 wurden 51 Kinder und Jugendliche im Alter von 5–18 Jahren wegen Schilddrüsenerkrankungen operiert, darunter 42 mit benignen Schilddrüsenerkrankungen (juvenile Struma 21, Adenome 17, Basedow-Struma 3, Hashimoto-Thyreoiditis 1) and 9 mit Malignomen (papilläre Karzinome 4, follikuläre Karzinome 3, medulläres Karzinom 1, undifferenziertes Karzinom 1). Bei den benignen Erkrankungen waren Mädchen 3mal häufiger betroffen als Jungen, bei den Malignomen war die Geschlechtsverteilung gleich. Eine positive Familienanamnese fand sich bei 23,3% der Kinder mit Adenomen und bei 71,4% der Kinder mit juveniler Struma; 30mal wurde eine subtotale Strumektomie und 12mal eine Enukleation durchgeführt. Jodiertes Speisesalz und L-Thyroxin wurden zur postoperativen Rezidivprophylaxe gegeben. Bei 2 Kindern, die keine Rezidivprophylaxe durchgeführt hatten, kam es zum Strumarezidiv (4,8%).

Erstsymptome bei Kindern mit Schilddrüsenmalignomen waren tastbare Halslymphknoten und Solitärknoten in der Schilddrüse. Totale Thyreoidektomien wurden in allen Fällen vorgenommen. 8 Kinder wurden postoperativ mit Radiojod behandelt, und bei einem Kind wurde eine ^{60}Co-Bestrahlung durchgeführt. 2 Kinder starben an diffuser Metastasierung bzw. Strahlenfibrose der Lunge.

Die Besonderheiten der chirurgischen Schilddrüsenerkrankungen im Kindesalter werden diskutiert.

[1] Pediatric Surgical Clinic and [2] Pediatric Clinic, Dr. von Haunersches Kinderspital of the University of Munich, Lindwurmstraße 4, D-8000 Munich 2 (W) FRG.

Progress in Pediatric Surgery, Vol. 26
Gauderer and Angerpointner (Eds.)
© Springer-Verlag Berlin Heidelberg 1991

Résumé

Entre 1970 et 1986, 51 enfants et adolescents, âgés de 5 à 18 ans ont été opérés pour une affection de la glande thyroïde; 42d'entre eux présentaient des affections bénignes (goitre juvénile: 21; adénome: 17; maladie de Basedow: 3; thyroïdite de Hashimoto: 1) et 9 des affections malignes (carcinome papillaire: 4; carcinome folliculaire: 3; carcinome médulaire: 1; carcinome ana-plasique: 1). Dans les cas bénins, il y avait trois fois plus de patientes que de patients alors que les deux sexes étaient représentés dans la même proportion dans les cas malins. Dans 23.3% des cas d'adénomes et 71.4% des cas de goitres juvéniles on note une prédisposition familiale. Dans 30 cas, on pratiqua une strumectomie subtotale et dans 12 cas une énucléation. On administra du sel iodé et de la thyroxine L(?) après l'intervention pour éviter une récurrence. Il y eut récurrence dans le cas de deux enfants qui avaient ignoré les mesures prophylactiques.

Les symptômes des affections malignes étaient les nodules lymphatiques cervicaux et les nodules solitaires de la glande thyroïde. Dans tous les cas, une thyroïdectomie totale a été pra-tiquée, suivie d'un traitement à l'iode radioactif dans 8 cas et d'irradiation au cobalt 60 dans un cas. Deux enfants sont décédés à la suite de métastases diffuses dans un cas et à une fibrose pul-monaire due à l'irradiation dans l'autre cas.

Suit une discussion sur les affections de la thyroïde relevant de la chirurgie des enfants.

Introduction

Juvenile, euthyroid, noninflammatory hyperplasia of the thyroid gland is the most common thyroid disease in childhood and adolescence. In some struma-endemic regions of Southern Germany, up to 10% of adolescents present with juvenile struma even today [13]. All other disorders of the thyroid gland, such as solitary nodules, immune thyroiditis, and hyper- and hypothyroidism are much rarer in children than in adults. Thus, every nodular goiter and, in particular, every soli-tary node that occurs in a child is more to be suspected of thyroid cancer than one occurring in an adult [9, 13, 21, 27].

Except for autonomous adenoma and thyroid cancer, diseases of the thyroid gland are primarily the domain of the pediatrician and the pediatric endocrinolo-gist [17]. Since the thyroid plays an essential role in the mental and somatic deve-lopment of children, special therapeutic principles must be followed in pediatric thyroid diseases.

According to Röher [23], surgical treatment is indicated if:

- The juvenile goiter is of extraordinary size (struma grade III) and sufficient re-gression with conservative treatment cannot be expected
- Tracheal and esophageal stenosis or venous blockage occurs
- There is a retrosternal struma
- Conservative treatment of even a minor goiter remains unsuccessful for 2 or more years
- The TSH-thyroid axis is disrupted (autonomous adenoma)
- Thyroid cancer is suspected

We present and discuss our patients with pediatric thyroid diseases who were sur-gically treated during the past two decades.

Patients

From 1970 through 1986, 51 children and adolescents aged 5–18 years were operated on for thyroid diseases at the Pediatric Surgical Clinic, Dr. von Haunersches
Kinderspital, of the University of Munich, 42 of them with benign and nine with
malignant entities.

Benign Diseases

Pathohistological examination of the 42 children with benign thyroid diseases revealed struma colloides in 21, adenoma in 17, Graves' disease in three and Hashimoto's thyroiditis in one (Table 1). There was a marked female preponderance,
with 31 girls and 11 boys, giving a sex ratio of 2.8:1.

Hereditary influences were evident with positive family histories in four children with adenomas (23.5%) and 15 children with struma colloides (71.4%). The
average age of the children was 12.5 years, with a range of 8–18 years. The average time span between appearance of first symptoms and operation was 2.1 years;
however, it was considerably shorter in adenoma than in struma colloides.

Surgically, subtotal strumectomy was carried out in 30 cases and enucleation
in 12 cases. Enucleation of an adenoma is the method of choice whenever the adenoma is sufficiently demarcated against the surrounding tissue.

Seven of the 42 children (16.7%) suffered postoperative complications (paralysis of the recurrent nerve, 2; reversible hypocalcemia, 1; wound-healing distur-
bances, 4). There was no death in the series.

Thirty-three of the 42 children with benign thyroid diseases were regularly re-
examined in our outpatient department. The remaining children were lost to follow-up. The average follow-up time was 4.2 years. There were no recurrences in
cases where recurrence prophylaxis with iodized table salt and L-thyroxine was regularly followed. However, two children (4.8%) developed a struma relapse, 7
and 9 years following surgery respectively. One child had been operated on for
struma colloides and the other for trabecular adenoma. Both children had not taken their recurrence prophylaxis.

Table 1. Benign thyroid diseases

Disease	Patients				
	n	Female	Male	Sex ratio	Positive family history
Struma colloides	21	16	5	3.2:1	15 (71.4%)
Adenoma	17	12	5	2.4:1	4 (23.5%)
Graves' disease	3	2	1		
Hashimoto's thyroiditis	1	1	–		
Total	42	31	11	2.8:1	

All children were prescribed a recurrence prophylaxis postoperatively. In a struma-endemic area, first the exogenous noxa, i.e., iodine deficiency, has to be eliminated; thus, all children were urged to use iodized table salt exclusively. Second, suppression of thyrotropin is mandatory to avoid a struma relapse. L-thyroxine, at a dose of 100 µg per day, proved to be useful as standard medication in children and adolescents to regulate-thyroid function. Children who had been operated on for adenoma were also given this recurrence prophylaxis.

Thyroid Cancer

Nine of the 52 children had to undergo surgery for thyroid cancer. Pathohistological examination revealed papillary carcinoma in four cases, follicular carcinoma in three cases, medullary (C-cell cancer) in one case and anaplastic carcinoma in the remaining case. The child with C-cell cancer suffered from the multiple endocrine neoplasia syndrome (MEN type IIb). Sex ratio was equal, with five girls and four boys (Table 2).

First symptoms in children with thyroid cancer were enlarged cervical lymph nodes and solitary nodules in the thyroid gland. Anamnestically, there was no preceding irradiation of the neck or the mediastinum. All children underwent total thyroidectomy in order not to endanger the relatively good prognosis in this age group by a less radical procedure. Total thyroidectomy was performed primarily in six cases and as a second-look procedure in the remaining three cases when the diagnosis was finally established by pathohistological examination. The affected cervical lymph nodes were surgically removed in seven cases, but no radical neck dissection was carried out.

Three of the nine children developed postoperative complications (paralysis of the recurrent nerve, Horner's syndrome, hypocalcemia). All children received substitution therapy with thyroid hormones postoperatively. Eight children underwent postoperative radioiodine treatment at a dose of 100–150 mCi for 1 month following surgery. One child with anaplastic carcinoma received ^{60}Co irradiation of the neck, axilla and mediastinum. This child died 2 months postoperatively of diffuse metastases including the myocardium. Another child with follicular carcinoma died 5 months postoperatively of lung fibrosis and irradiation pneumonitis. Thus, the survival rate in our series was 77.8%.

Table 2. Thyroid cancer

Histological type	Patients			
	n	Female	Male	Death
Papillary carcinoma	4	3	1	–
Follicular carcinoma	3	1	2	1
Medullary carcinoma (C-cell)	1	–	1	–
Anaplastic carcinoma	1	1	–	1
Total	9	5	4	2 (22.2%)

Discussion

Iodine deficiency is the etiologic agent for juvenile struma, effecting an increase in TSH [6, 24]. Surgery is indicated for juvenile struma if compression signs occur or if conservative treatment remains unsuccessful for a longer period of time. The Federal Republic of Germany is a struma-endemic country with a marked north-south gradient, the incidence being 4% in Schleswig-Holstein and 32% in Bavaria [16]. In the USA, in contrast, the incidence of juvenile struma is 1.8% [2].

The pronounced female predominance of up to 4.5:1 [14, 15, 17] was confirmed in our series. We have also found a very distinct hereditary component, with a positive family history of juvenile struma in 71% and of adenoma in 24%. Thus, exogenic and endogenic (hereditary) factors cooperate in the etiology of benign thyroid diseases in children and adolescents. Lindinger and Sitzmann [16] reported a struma incidence of 40% in the offspring if one parent had a struma and of 64% if both parents were affected.

Sufficiently iodized table salt available for everybody is very desirable for general prophylaxis in struma-endemic areas. In Switzerland, Austria, and Finland, the struma incidence was lowered to 3% by table salt iodization [14, 24, 25]. In the Federal Republic of Germany, sufficiently iodized table salt (100 µg iodine per 5 g salt) has been available since 1982 [24], but its use is still voluntary.

Since the same etiologic factors remain active postoperatively, the necessity of postoperative recurrence prophylaxis with L-thyroxine and iodized table salt is generally accepted [3, 4, 7, 15, 23, 26]. The principle is depression of the TSH axis. Prior to the introduction of postoperative recurrence prophylaxis, the recurrence rate was 60% secondary to subtotal strumectomy [3]. Today, postoperative struma recurrence is reported to be from 1.2% up to 10%, with a mean incidence of 5% [3, 7, 15, 23, 26], which is in good accordance with our recurrence rate of 4.8%. Most authors, however, emphasize that the majority of recurrences are seen in patients who disregard the prophylactic treatment, as was the case with our two patients who developed struma relapse postoperatively. Bartels et al. [3] stressed that after 2 years only 60% of patients take their prophylaxis regularly. Permanent prophylaxis with L-thyroxine and iodized table salt securely prevents struma relapse.

Thyroid autonomy is the excess production of thyroid hormones without hypophyseal influence via TSH regulation. The treatment of choice is surgery, with enucleation of the adenoma if it is sufficiently demarcated against the surrounding tissue. If this is not the case, subtotal strumectomy has to be carried out [7, 11, 17, 20, 23, 27]. We gave recurrence prophylaxis also after surgery for thyroid adenoma. Since the etiology of adenoma is still not completely clear, no general agreement on postoperative recurrence prophylaxis exists in the literature. However, the fact that one of our patients with an adenoma who did not take L-thyroxine postoperatively developed a relapse is a hint at the usefulness of postoperative recurrence prophylaxis also in adenoma. We are of the opinion that in a struma-endemic region the depression of the TSH axis may also prevent a relapse of an adenoma.

The largest series of childhood thyroid cancer in the German-speaking countries was published by Joppich et al. in 1980 [10]. It included 25 children examined in a multicenter study. Thyroid cancer occurs in 1% of all malignomas, whereby every 20th patient is a child; thus it is the most common carcinoma in childhood [10, 21]. In comparison with adults, thyroid cancer in childhood presents very often (up to 70%) with enlarged cervical lymph nodes as the initial symptom [1, 2, 8–10, 12, 14, 21, 22]. Reiter et al. [22] even speak of primary lymph node metastases in 85% of children with thyroid carcinoma. Scintigraphically cold nodes in children are much more to be suspected of thyroid cancer than in adults [8–10, 13, 14, 17, 21]. Thus, according to Reiter et al. [22], cold nodules are malignant in 17%–40% of cases, in even 60% of cases (vs. 13% in adults) according to Herzog [8]. Every cold nodule must therefore be excised [18]. Thyroid cancer often develops secondary to irradiation of the neck and the mediastinum [17, 21]. However, almost all thyroid cancers in childhood are well differentiated [1, 27]. Papillary carcinoma with a very favorable prognosis predominates in this age-group, followed by follicular carcinoma with a little less favorable but still good prognosis [9, 10, 17, 23]. Medullary (C-cell) carcinoma and anaplastic carcinoma with poor prognoses fortunately play a minor role in childhood [5].

The good overall prognosis of childhood thyroid cancer with a cure rate of 80%–90% [1, 8, 17, 27], which is in accordance with our figures, however, leads to a controversial discussion on surgical radicality in the literature. One group of authors favor a less radical surgical procedure (lobectomy, subtotal strumectomy, enucleation) because of the good prognosis [2, 8, 14, 18], whereas a second, larger group of authors favor total, radical thyroidectomy with surgical removal of the affected cervical lymph nodes. They argue that in 30%–80% of cases an intraglandular tumor dissemination affects the contralateral part of the thyroid [1, 5, 9, 10, 17, 19, 21, 23, 26, 27]. Together with this latter group, we are of the opinion that the favorable prognosis of childhood thyroid cancer must not be endangered by a less radical surgical procedure. We therefore recommend total thyroidectomy with excision of the affected cervical lymph nodes; this was done in all our patients with thyroid cancer. A 90% survival rate may be achieved by applying all therapeutic measures such as surgery, radioiodine treatment, hormone substitution and, in special cases, external irradiation.

Conclusion

The variety of thyroid disorders in childhood and adolescence, both benign and malignant, requires a very consistent therapeutic regime because of the special tasks of the thyroid gland in this age-group. Close cooperation between pediatricians, pediatric endocrinologists and pediatric surgeons is mandatory to ensure a good to excellent prognosis in benign as well as in malignant diseases.

References

1. Anger K, Feine U (1983) Thyroid carcinoma in childhood. Prog Pediatr Surg 16:39–42
2. Balazs G, Lukacs G, Csaky G, Boros P, Ilyes J (1986) Spätergebnisse kindlicher Schilddrüsenkarzinome. Presented at the 5th ACE Meeting, Hamburg, Sept 19/20
3. Bartels H, Erdt E, Haluszczynski I (1982) Sind Rezidive nach Resektionen benigner Schilddrüsenerkrankungen vermeidbar? Fortschr Med 82:1108–1110
4. Benker G (1986) Diagnostik und Therapiekontrolle bei M. Basedow. Therapiewoche 36: 1724–1730
5. Bindewald H, Raue F, Merkle P (1983) The diagnosis and therapy of medullary thyroid carcinoma in childhood. Prog Pediatr Surg 16:43–46
6. Butenandt O (1983) Die Therapie endokriner Erkrankungen im Kindes- und Jugendlichenalter. Fortschr Med 101:667–669
7. Csaky G, Balazs G, Bako G, Ilyes J, Kalman K, Szabo J (1986) Spätresultate der im Kindesalter durchgeführten Schilddrüsenoperationen wegen Hyperthyreose. Presented at the 5th ACE Meeting, Hamburg, Sept 19/20
8. Herzog B (1983) Thyroid gland diseases and tumors – surgical aspects. Prog Pediatr Surg 16:15–22
9. Joppich I, Röher HD, Hecker WC, Knorr D, Daum R (1980) Besonderheiten des Schilddrüsenkarzinomes im Kindesalter. Klin Padiatr 192:436–439
10. Joppich I, Röher HD, Hecker WC, Knorr D, Daum R (1983) Thyroid carcinoma in childhood. Prog Pediatr Surg 16:23–27
11. Joseph K (1986) Thyreoidale Autonomie. Therapiewoche 36:1711–1723
12. Kaiser P, Wurnig P (1980) Seltene Erkrankungen der kindlichen Schilddrüse. Z Kinderchir 30:112–114
13. Klein E, Blaeser W (1969) Die Therapie der juvenilen Struma. Dtsch Med Wochenschr 94:609–611
14. Ladurner D, Riccabona G (1986) Schilddrüsenerkrankungen im Kindesalter aus chirurgischer Sicht. Presented at the 5th ACE Meeting, Hamburg, Sept 19/20
15. Langenbach J (1986) Zehn Jahre Schilddrüsenchirurgie. Therapiewoche 36:2336–2342
16. Lindinger A, Sitzmann C (1978) Die juvenile Struma. Kinderarzt 9:277–281
17. Nüllen H, Sailer R, Müller E (1979) Chirurgie der Schilddrüse im Kindesalter. Kinderarzt 10:1129–1134
18. Pfister-Goedeke L, Stauffer UG (1983) Thyroid carcinoma in childhood. Prog Pediatr Surg 16:29–37
19. Pohl P (1983) Schilddrüsenchirurgie. In: Heberer G, Köle W, Tscherne H (eds) Chirurgie. Springer, Berlin Heidelberg New York, pp 440–448
20. Rauh V, Kujath HP, Reimers C, Höcht B (1989) Indikation, operative Therapie und Nachsorge bei der kindlichen Hyperthyreose. Presented at the 5th ACE Meeting, Hamburg, Sept 19/20
21. Ravitch MM (1979) The thyroid. In: Ravitch MM, Welch KJ, Benson CD, Aberdeen E, Randolph JG (eds) Pediatric surgery.. Yearbook Med Publ Mediat, Chicago, pp 348–364
22. Reiter EO, Root AW, Rettig K (1981) Childhood thyromegaly: recent developments. J Pediatr 99:507–518
23. Röher H-D (1987) Endokrine Chirurgie. Thieme, Stuttgart, pp 1–35
24. Scriba PC (1983) Pathophysiologie der blanden Struma und Jodsalzprophylaxe. Therapiewoche 32:29–34
25. Wiebei J (1981) Die sogenannte euthyreote Struma im Kindes- und Jugendlichenalter. Kinderarzt 12:1411–1413
26. Waag K-L, Hanisch E, Kollmann F, Wons T, Wenisch H (1988) Erfahrung mit der operativen Therapie von Schilddrüsenerkrankungen im Kindesalter. Z Kinderchir 43:232–235
27. Zabransky S (1983) Seltene Schilddrüsenerkrankungen im Kindesalter. Therapiewoche 33:61–72

Indications, Surgical Treatment and After-Care in Juvenile Hyperthyroidism

V. Rauh[1], H. P. Kujath[1], C. Reimers[2], and B. Höcht[1]

Summary

Between 1974 and 1985, 12 children and adolescents aged 10–18 years were operated on for immunogenic hyperthyroidism resistant to medical treatment. Bilateral, subtotal strumectomies were carried out, leaving a remnant of 2–3 g of thyroid tissue in place. There were no immediate postoperative complications. Hyperthyroidism recurred in two instances. During the same time, 26 children and adolescents up to 18 years of age underwent surgery for autonomous adenoma. Enucleation is the method of choice in adenoma, but is not always possible.

Zusammenfassung

Von 1974 bis 1985 wurden 12 Kinder und Heranwachsende im Alter von 10–18 Jahren wegen einer therapieresistenten Hyperthyreose operiert. Dabei wurde eine bilaterale, subtotale Strumektomie mit einem Schilddrüsenrest von 2–3 g durchgeführt. Unmittelbare postoperative Komplikationen wurden nicht beobachtet. Zu einem Hyperthyreoserezidiv kam es in 2 Fällen. Im gleichen Zeitraum wurden 26 Kinder und Jugendliche bis 18 Jahre wegen eines autonomen Adenoms operiert. Die Enukleation ist das Verfahren der Wahl, jedoch nicht immer durchführbar.

Résumé

Entre 1974 et 1985, 12 enfants et adolescents âgés de 10 à 18 ans ont été opérés pour hyperthyréose immunogénétiques résistant au traitement médical. Des strumectomies bilatérales et subtotales ont été pratiquées, laissant en place un reste de 2 à 3 g de tissu thyroïdien. Il n'y a pas eu de complications postopératoires. Dans deux cas, il y a eu récurrence de l'hyperthyréose. Au cours de la même période, 26 enfants et adolescents (âge maximum: 18 ans) ont subi une intervention chirurgicale pour adénome autonome. Si l'énucléation reste la méthode de choix, elle n'est malheureusement pas toujours possible.

Treatment of hyperthyroidism relies on three main supports:

1. Medical therapy (thyrostatic drugs, hormone substitution, iodine treatment)
2. Surgical removal of thyroid tissue
3. Radioiodine therapy

Radioiodine therapy for benign thyroid diseases is contraindicated in childhood and adolescence because of possible induction of malignancy. The other two

[1]University Surgical Clinic of Würzburg and [2]Department of Nuclear Medicine, University of Würzburg, Josef-Schneider-Straße 2, D-8700 Würzburg (W), FRG.

Table 1. Additional findings in immunogenic
hyperthyroid struma (1974–1985; $n = 12$; age
10–18 years)

Chronic lymphocytic thyroiditis (Hashimoto)	6 (50%!)
Further autoimmune diseases (such as myasthenia gravis)	1
Endocrine ophthalmopathy	6
Preoperative thyrotoxic crisis	1

therapies do not compete with each other, but rather have their own clear indications:

- Early operation is desirable for a child with nonimmunogenic hyperthyroidism, such as autonomous adenoma.
- Medical treatment is the primary step in diffuse immunogenic, hyperthyroid struma (Graves' disease) in children.

We use carbimazole as the primary thyrostatic drug. If euthyroidism cannot be achieved after 6 weeks, L-thyroxine is given in addition. If medical treatment is unsuccessful for a longer period of time, i.e., at least 2 years, surgery is indicated.

Between 1974 and 1985, 12 children aged between 10 and 18 years were operated on for immunogenic hyperthyroid struma resistant to medical therapy at the University Surgical Hospital of Würzburg, among a total of 137 operations for benign thyroid diseases. Medical therapy lasted 2.75 years on the average, ranging from 6 months to 5 years. Additional findings are shown in Table 1

Besides unsuccessful medical therapy, further indications for surgery are:

- Insufficient cooperation on the part of the patient
- Displacement of surrounding structures by the struma
- Recurrent hyperthyroidism following surgery leading to regressive changes (cold nodules)

If there are no regressive changes, recurrent hyperthyroidism is treated primarily with thyrostatic drugs in childhood.

Postoperative hyperthyroidism must be regarded as failure of treatment. In contrast, postoperative hypothyroidism can be easily controlled by hormone substitution. However, it must be kept in mind that immunogenic hyperthyroidism usually ends in hypothyroidism.

By means of preoperative administration of thyrostatic drugs and L-thyroxine, all 12 children had normal thyroid function prior to surgery. Bilateral, subtotal strumectomies were performed for immunogenic hyperthyroidism. Thus the inferior thyroid artery is left intact; the recurrent nerve is not exhibited routinely. A remnant of 2–3 g of thyroid tissue per side is desirable.

Table 2. Preoperative thyroid metabolism in autonomous adenoma (1974–1985; $n = 26$; age 10–18 years)

Compensated	16
thereof normal	10
hyperthyroid	6
Decompensated	10
thereof normal	4
hyperthyroid	6

Table 3. Surgical procedures in children and adolescents (1974–1985; $n = 38$; age 10–18 years)

Immunogenic hyperthyroid struma ($n = 12$)	
bilateral subtotal resection	12
Autonomous adenoma ($n = 26$)	
Enucleation	9
Unilateral subtotal resection	11
Bilateral subtotal resection	6

There were no immediate postoperative complications such as permanent paralysis of the recurrent nerve, hypoparathyroidism or postoperative thyrotoxic crisis. We did not employ medical therapy routinely postoperatively. This depended on the findings at the first follow-up, 4–5 weeks following surgery, enabling an adequate drug therapy. At follow-up we found hypothyroid metabolism in six cases. Two children developed recurrent hyperthyroidism within 1 year of surgery.

Autonomous adenomas are rare in childhood. During the same time period we operated on 26 children and adolescents up to 18 years of age. The youngest patient was 10, most patients were older than 15 years (mean 16.7 years).

Preoperative thyroid metabolism is shown in Table 2 and operative procedures applied are presented in Table 3. Surgery was carried out as soon as normal thyroid function was achieved (about 6 weeks after establishment of diagnosis). Enucleation must be considered the method of choice in autonomous adenoma. However, we were able to perform it could be carried in only nine of the 26 patients. Unilateral subtotal resection was performed in 11 cases and bilateral subtotal resection in six. This was due to paranodular changes of the thyroid tissue, i.e., a multifocal struma. Nuclear medical follow-up revealed normal thyroid metabolism in 14 cases and hypothyroid metabolism in 12.

References

1. Bay V, Engel U (1980) Komplikationen bei Schilddrüsenoperationen. Chirurg 51:91–98
2. Butenandt O (1983) Die Therapie endokriner Erkrankungen im Kindes- und Jugendalter. Fortschr Med 15:665–716
3. Helbig D (1974) Schilddrüsenchirurgie im Kindesalter. Münch Med Wochenschr 116:1139–1142
4. Koch B, Wilker D (1982) Prä- und postoperative Therapie der Hyperthyreose. Dtsch Med Wochenschr 107:1519–1520
5. Schumann J, Grabs V (1975) Zur Problematik der subtotalen Strumaresektion bei Hyperthyreose mit endokriner Ophthalmopathie. Langenbecks Arch Chir 338:251–263
6. Stubbe P, Heidemann P, Droese M, Schatz H, Kaboth U (1984) Schilddrüsenerkrankungen im Kindes- und Adoleszentenalter. Münch Med Wochenschr 126:857–860
7. Wesley JR et al. (1977) Surgical treatment of hyperthyroidism in children. Surg Gynecol Obstet 145:344–346

Late Results of Thyroid Surgery
for Hyperthyroidism Performed in Childhood

G. Csáky[1], G. Balázs[2], G. Bakó[3], I. Ilyés[4], K. Kálmán[3], and J. Szabó[3]

Summary

The authors report on the complex follow-up of 60 patients operated on for hyperthyroidism in childhood, on average 13.7 years after surgery. In 16.7% of the patients manifest hypothyroidism, in 45% subclinical hypothyroidism was found; 30% of the patients were euthyroid, and manifest hyperthyroidism recurred in 8.3%. Autonomous adenomas were enucleated in two children and three young adults.

Severe disorders in thyroid function developed especially after the surgery of diffuse toxic goiters accompanied by ophthalmopathy. The disorders of humoral and cellular immunity were detected most frequently in recurrent manifest hyperthyroidism. There was no case where ophthalmopathy progressed after the operation.

In the offspring of the operated patients the incidence of hyperthyroidism was not increased in childhood. The authors call attention to the importance of postoperative follow-up and hormone treatment.

Zusammenfassung

Es wird über die Ergebnisse von Nachuntersuchungen bei 60 Patienten berichtet, die wegen einer Hyperthyreose operiert worden waren. Die Untersuchungen fanden im Durchschnitt 13,7 Jahre nach der Operation statt. Bei 16,7% wurde eine manifeste und bei 45% eine subklinische Hypothyreose gefunden, wogegen 30% der Patienten euthyreot waren und 8,3% eine manifeste Hyperthyreose aufwiesen. Autonome Adenome wurden bei 2 Kindern und 3 jungen Erwachsenen enukleiert.

Schwere Störungen der Schilddrüsenfunktion traten v.a. nach Operationen diffuser, toxischer Strumen mit begleitender Ophthalmopathie auf. Störungen der humoralen und zellulären Immunität wurden meist bei rezidivierender manifester Hyperthyreose gefunden. In keinem Fall kam es postoperativ zur Progredienz der Ophthalmopathie.

Bei den Kindern der operierten Patienten war die Häufigkeit einer Hyperthyreose gegenüber anderen Kindern nicht erhöht. Es wird nachdrücklich auf die Notwendigkeit der postoperativen Nachuntersuchungen und der Hormonsubstitution hingewiesen.

Résumé

Les auteurs ont suivi, de façon très complexe, pendant une moyenne de 13,7 ans après l'opération 60 patients ayant subi durant leur enfance une intervention chirurgicale pour hyperthyroïdie.

[1] Department of Surgery, County Hospital, 3501 Miskolc, Hungary.
[2] First Clinic of Surgery,
[3] First Clinic of Medicine, and [4] Clinic of Pediatrics of the University Medical School, POB 27, 4012 Debrecen, Hungary.

Progress in Pediatric Surgery, Vol. 26
Gauderer and Angerpointner (Eds.)
© Springer-Verlag Berlin Heidelberg 1991

Chez 16,7% des patients on note une hypothyroïdie manifeste, une hypothyroïdie subclinique chez 45%, une euthyroïdie chez 30%, une récurrence d'hyperthyroïdie manifeste chez 8,3%. On a pratiqué l'énucléation d'un adénome autonome chez deux enfants et trois jeunes adultes.

Des troubles graves de la fonction thyroïdienne sont apparus surtout après l'ablation chirurgicale de goitres diffus toxiques accompagnés d'ophtalmopathie. Les troubles de l'immunité humorale et cellulaire sont plus fréquents dans les cas de récurrence d'une hyperthyroïdie manifeste. Après l'intervention on ne constate aucun cas d'évolution de l'ophtalmopathie.

Chez les enfants des patients ayant subi une intervention, on ne constate pas, durant l'enfance, une augmentation de la fréquence de l'hyperthyroïdie. Les auteurs insistent sur l'importance du suivi postopératoire et du traitement hormonal.

Introduction

The most frequent cause of thyroid hyperfunction in childhood is immune hyperthyroidism associated with the diffuse enlargement of the thyroid gland. In comparison with adult cases nodular lesions are less common, and ophthalmopathy has a more favourable prognosis. Since after 1–3 years of antithyroid drug treatment hyperthyroidism recurs in 40%–70% of cases, several authors [14, 31] prefer surgical intervention, others [12, 24] radioiodine therapy in childhood and adolescence.

At present we have only a few data on the late results of thyroid surgery for childhood hyperthyroidism, e.g., on postoperative thyroid function, humoral and cellular immunological changes, and the childhood thyroid diseases of the progeny. Therefore, we consider it worthwhile to make our investigations in this field public.

Methods and Materials

At the First Clinic of Surgery of the University Medical School of Debrecen between 1951 and 1980, 68 operations were performed on patients under 18 years of age for hyperthyroidism. In the 1950s, for the establishment of the diagnosis we used, besides the clinical picture, the basal metabolic test, serum cholesterol and PBI determinations; later ^{131}I uptake, thyroid scan, and suppression tests; and in the last 15 years of the period under discussion thyroid hormone assay and TRH-TSH test.

The thyroid lobes that were diffusely or nodularly transformed on both sides were subtotally resected after preparation with antithyroid drugs and Lugol's solution, and 6–10 g of thyroid tissue was retained. Autonomous adenomas were enucleated. The patients who underwent postoperative thyroid hormone treatment stopped taking the medicine 2 weeks before the follow-up examination.

Of the 68 operated patients, 60 were re-examined in 1984, an average of 13.7 years after surgery. During the re-examination the following tests were performed on the patients' sera: T_4-RIA (our own laboratory, norm 55–155 nmol/l), T_3-RIA (our own laboratory, norm 1.6–3.4 nmol/l) and T_3 uptake (our own laboratory, norm 0.85–1.15). In addition, TRH-loading tests were performed with the i.v.

administration of 200 μg TRH (Berlin-Chemie) (ΔTSH: 20' TSH–0' TSH mU/l) (TSH-RIA, Byk-Mallinckrodt, norm: 0.6–3.8 mU/l). From the product of the T_3-uptake and T_4-RIA results, FT_4I (norm: 60–160), and from the product of T_3 uptake and T_3-RIA, FT_3I (norm: 1.3–3.5) were calculated. On the basis of the hormone assays the patients were classified into four groups (manifest and subclinical hypothyroidism, euthyroidism and manifest hyperthyroidism). The anti-human-thyroglobulin and anti-microsomal antibody titres were determined by the Boyden [4] passive haemagglutination method. The upper limit of normal agglutination values was 1:16. According to the procedure of Roitt and Doniach [23], the presence of the anti-thyroglobulin and anti-microsomal antibodies was also examined by the indirect immunofluorescence method using FITC-labelled anti-human-IgG (Hyland). The location, character and intensity of fluorescence were evaluated [28]. To determine cellular immunity, leucocyte migration tests were performed [17]:

$$\text{migration index} = \frac{\text{migration area with the presence of antigen}}{\text{migration area without antigen}}.$$

(norm: 0.8–1.2). The anti-TSH receptor antibody was detected in the sera of the re-examined patients by the dot-immunobinding assay [15]. The reactions distinguished were: positive (+), negative (−) and uncertain positive (+). The ophthalmological symptoms were classified with Werner's method [30]. The functioning of the vocal cords was checked. Of 79 children of the operated patients 40 were examined, and if there was suspicion of a thyroid disease hormone assays were carried out. The statistical analysis was performed with Student's t-test.

Results

The thyroid enlargement and the hyperthyroid symptoms in the 60 (re-examined) patients began 1.8 years before surgery on the average. The majority of the symptoms consisted in neurological (psychic) disorders and tachycardia. The surgical indication was given in the case of 15 patients by ineffective antithyroid treatment for an average of 1.3 years. Medicine-induced toxic side effects or leucopenia necessitated the termination of medicinal treatment in 11 patients. The surgical solution was imperative in three cases because of insufficient cooperation. In the other cases the largeness of the goitre or its nodular character indicated the operation. The average age of the patients at the time of the operation was 15.6 years (the youngest was 10). The autonomous adenoma proved to be decompensated in two cases and compensated in three. Detailed histological examination revealed more pronounced than usual instances of associated lymphocytic thyroiditis in nine cases. No postoperative thyrotoxic crisis or hypoparathyroidism was observed. There was only one case in which final unilateral paresis of the recurrent nerve developed.

Table 1 summarizes the distribution of thyroid functions according to preoperative diagnosis, as observed at follow-up and from the results of the hor-

Table 1. Thyroid function of patients operated on for hyperthyroidism: diagnosis at surgery compared with follow-up hormone assay data

Diagnosis at surgery	Manifest hypothyroidism (No. of cases)	Subclinical hypothyroidism (No. of cases)	Euthyroidism (No. of cases)	Manifest hyperthyroidism (No. of cases)
Autonomous adenoma $n = 5$	–	–	5	–
Multinodular toxic goitre $n = 9$	1	4	4	–
Diffuse toxic goitre				
A: without ophthalmopathy $n = 19$	2	10	6	1
B: with ophthalmopathy $n = 27$	7	13	3	4
Total $n = 60$ (100%)	10 (16.7%)	27 (45%)	18 (30%)	5 (8.3%)
Hormone assay	Mean ± SEM	Mean ± SEM	Mean ± SEM	Mean ± SEM
FT_3I	1.43 ± 0.70	2.09 ± 0.53	2.36 ± 0.65	5.33 ± 2.22
FT_4I	48.5 ± 12.1	83.6 ± 24.4	94.0 ± 20.4	186 ± 50.2
TSH 0' (mU/l)	24.6 ± 22.3	8.57 ± 5.40	2.49 ± 0.87	1.13 ± 0.27
ΔTSH (mU/l)	50.5 ± 17.5	39.0 ± 19.8	12.5 ± 6.5	0

Not significant

N.S.

N.S.

N.S.

Table 2. Thyroid function of patients operated on for hyperthyroidism: immunological assay data at follow-up according to diagnosis at surgery

Diagnosis at surgery	Manifest hypothyroidism DOT-IBA n	+	+−	IF Tg+	Mi+	Subclinical hypothyroidism DOT-IBA n	+	+−	IF Tg+	Mi+	Euthyroidism DOT-IBA n	+	+−	IF Tg+	Mi+	Manifest hyperthyroidism DOT-IBA n	+	+−	IF Tg+	Mi+
Autonomous adenoma (n = 5)	—					—					5		1			—				
Hyperfunctional multinodular goitre (n = 9)	1		1			4	1	2	1	1	4			1	1	—				
Hyperfunctional diffuse goitre A: without ophthalmopathy (n = 19)	2					10		1	2		6	2			2	1			1	
B: with ophthalmopathy	7	1		2	3	13	1	2	2	3	3	1		1		4	3		1	
Total (n = 60)	10 (16.7%)	1	1	2	3	27 (45%)	2	5	5	4	18 (30%)	3	1	2	3	5 (8.3%)	3		2	

DOT-IBA, Dot-immunobinding-assay + (positive), +− (uncertain positive); IF, indirect immunofluorescence: Tg+ (anti-thyroglobulin antibody: positive), Mi+ (anti-microsome antibody: positive)

mone assays. All patients operated on for autonomous adenoma became euthyroid. The late operative results for nine cases of hyperfunctional multinodular goitre are also good, since only one case of manifest hypothyroidism was found. Of the four patients who became euthyroid, one had hyperplasia of the pyramidal lobe, one unilateral diffuse hypertrophy and one nodular recurrence. At the same time there was no recurrence of goitre among the four subclinical hypothyroid patients. Supposedly, the hypofunctional thyroid gland could compensate for the dysfunction through the development of recurrences. Recurring manifest hyperthyroidism was found only among those operated on for diffuse toxic goitre − the largest number among the cases complicated with ophthalmopathy −, and manifest hypothyroidism, too, occurred most frequently among these patients. Not included in the table are the significant differences in the hormone assay results forming the basis for group distribution.

In Table 2 the results of the immune assays are detailed. The anti-TSH receptor antibody serum assay gave positive results in three of five patients with manifest recurrent hyperthyroidism. In the other thyroid-functional groups anti-receptor antibodies were found relatively less frequently. With the method of indirect immunofluorescence anti-microsomal antibodies were found in the sera of 12 patients, anti-thyroglobulin antibodies in nine cases. Antibody positivity was relatively most frequently found in manifest hypothyroidism (in five of ten cases) and recurrent manifest hyperthyroidism (in two of five cases). At the same time, antibody positivity against both antigens was observed in none of the patients. In the group of those with manifest hypothyroidism there was no case at follow-up in which a rise in the titre was observed on antibody assay with Boyden's passive haemagglutination method. With the leucocyte migration test inhibition of migration was detected in seven patients against microsomal antigen and in five against thyroglobulin antigen. Inhibition of migration was proven in three patients against both thyroglobulin and microsomal antigen; two of them belonged to the subclinical hypothyroid, one to the manifest hypothyroid group. Inhibition of migration was detected against microsomal antigen in the sera of two of five patients with manifest recurrent hyperthyroidism. Summarizing the results of the immunological assays, one can establish that it is the patients with manifest recurrent hyperthyroidism in whom both humoral and cellular immunity remain defective after the operation. The disorders of immune regulation can be occasionally observed in the other functional groups, too; nevertheless, no closer connection can be proved statistically between the preoperative diagnosis, the later thyroid function and the positive results of the various immunological examinations.

There was remission of ophthalmopathy in 18 cases; in nine cases the condition became better or stationary (according to the ATA scale in two patients *1* on both eyes, in two patients *2a* on both eyes, and in five patients asymmetrically − *2a* on one eye and *1* on the other. Progression was not observed in any of the cases. Among the patients who still have ophthalmopathy, hyperthyroidism recurred in two; four developed manifest hypothyroidism and three subclinical hypothyroidism. Thus, it is obvious that the state of ophthalmopathy shows close correlation with thyroid function.

Thyroid surgery was repeated in three patients for recurrent hyperthyroid goitre 10, 10 and 11 years after the first surgical intervention. Radioiodine therapy was given to one patient for thyroid hyperfunction 2 years after the operation; however, this patient is hyperfunctional even now and is, at present, undergoing antithyroid treatment.

Among the children of the operated patients only one 22-year-old hyperfunctional female patient was found (without ophthalmopathy and goitre). The operation does not seem to adversely influence the fertility of women, and we do not have to reckon with an elevated frequency of hyperthyroidism among their offspring.

Discussion

The histological structure of the thyroid gland of children differs greatly from that of adults: for example, autonomous adenoma, hardly occurs in children and hyperfunctional nodular goitre is also much less frequent [21]. The appearance and course of some symptoms of hyperthyroidism are also different: there is a preponderance of lesions of the nervous system; on the other hand, ophthalmopathy is milder and has a better prognosis. The possibilities of therapy are also different, since radioiodine treatment is counterindicated in the opinion of a number of authors.

The majority of authors agree that in childhood hyperthyroidism can be treated successfully in 30%–60% of cases with antithyroid drugs [3, 14].

Nevertheless, the aim that the child become euthyroid in the shortest possible time with long-lasting results can be achieved in the rest of the cases only by surgical methods.

Abe and associates [1], also taking into account the previously published data, reported on 11 cases of childhood autonomous thyroid adenomas and found it characteristic that there was no connection between the size of the thyroid nodules of the children and the onset of their hyperthyroidism. Since the solitary nodule in childhood raises the suspicion of carcinoma, and this suspicion is not ruled out even by existing hyperthyroidism, in the treatment of autonomous adenoma enucleation is indicated. Among our patients with autonomous adenoma, the lesion of the two 13-year-old girls can be regarded as childhood disorders, whereas the autonomous adenoma in the three 17-year-old patients is rather to be evaluated as disease in early adulthood.

Whereas Saxena et al. [25], in the histopathological examination of 70 children with hyperthyroidism, found no more than four nodular disorders, Mäenpää und Kuusi [19] observed multinodular lesions in 11 cases of 40 in Finland. For their treatment hardly anything but surgery is recommended, since for nodular lesions lasting remission cannot be attained with antithyroid drugs. In the development of nodular goitre in our patients iodine deficiency may have played a role, our area being an endemic goitre district. In the course of the investigations on humoral immunity, in a striking way, several pathological cases were observed. This is suggestive of the possible role of immune globulins in the development of nodular goitres; on the other hand, it cannot be ruled out that disorders of different nature can occur contemporaneously or subsequently in the thyroid gland.

In children one can reckon with the development of hypothyroidism in 20 % – 60 % of cases after surgery for diffuse toxic goitre [6, 29]. The onset of the disorder in childhood is influenced, in a way similar to that in adults, by two factors: the amount of remaining thyroid tissue and the accompanying lymphocytic thyroiditis. The more thyroid tissue remains, the greater is the likelihood of recurrence of hyperthyroidism. In 12.7% of the 558 instances of operation for hyperthyroidism in childhood collected from the literature, hyperfunction of the thyroid gland recurred [21]. Some of the authors [12, 19] recommend radioiodine treatment in these cases even in childhood, since one has to reckon with more complications after repeated operations. To ensure prevention of recurrent hyperthyroidism, Perzik [22] recommends total thyroidectomy in childhood as the first surgical intervention; however, this view has not been adopted by the majority of surgeons.

Endocrine ophthalmopathy occurs in 50%–70% of children with hyperfunctional diffuse goitre [2, 20]. It is well known that, compared with adulthood, the symptoms are milder and mostly disappear when euthyroidism is attained. Deterioration after treatment was found in 1% of the patients by Barnes and Blizzard [3], and there was a difference in the extent of remission on the two sides in 37%.

Following thyroid surgery for Graves' disease, the amount of stimulating immunoglobulin and the titre of anti-thyroid antibodies decrease [26]. Finke et al. [11] invariably detected thyroid-stimulating antibody in 50% of the patients after thyroid operation; nevertheless, some of these patients became hypothyroid. These authors interpreted these results to indicate that because the mass of thyroid tissue was decreased due to the operation, the antibody could not cause thyroid hyperfunction. Lymphocytic infiltration of varying extent can be proved in 75% of the thyroid glands of patients with Graves' disease [9, 10]; it is accompanied by a lower degree of antibody titre elevation in the serum [27]. In Hashimoto's disease, in which lymphocytic thyroiditis and elevated anti-thyroid antibody titres are detected, one frequently finds thyroid hypofunction; therefore, we are justified in assuming that in the patients who become hypothyroid following surgery for Graves' disease, thyroid failure is due to the accompanying thyroiditis [32]. Surgery is favourable in thyroiditis only in view of the fact that by removing a given amount of antigen the pathological immunoprocesses are reduced [5]. Spontaneous inhibition of leucocyte migration was observed in Graves' disease, especially in the cases complicated by ophthalmopathy [18]. In the course of our investigations we found inhibition in the presence of the various antigens of the thyroid in the individual thyroid-functional groups, which indicates that the disorder of the genetically determined cellular immunoregulation can be proved even years after the operation, and it is not influenced by the concentration of the thyroid hormones.

The fact that in 17% of the patients manifest, and in 45% subclinical hypothyroidism was diagnosed emphasizes the importance of postoperative follow-up and hormone treatment. Regular checking of the patient's thyroid function seems to be necessary until the end of the patient's life. Thyroid hormone substitution is obligatory in manifest and subclinical hypothyroidism, whereas there are different opinions on hormone therapy in a euthyroid state [8, 16].

There are observations to suggest [7, 13] that both Graves' disease and Hashimoto's thyroiditis can occur in an accumulative way in a family. On the basis of our results we have established only that in the offspring of parents operated on in childhood for hyperthyroidism no higher rate of juvenile thyroid hyperfunction was found.

Abbreviations

PBI = Protein-bound iodine
TRH = Thyrotropin-releasing hormone
TSH = Thyroid-stimulating hormone
T_3 = Triiodothyronine
T_4 = Thyroxine
FT_3I = Free triiodothyronine index
FT_4I = Free thyroxine index
IgG = Immunoglobulin-G
ATA = American Thyroid Association

References

1. Abe K, Konno M, Sato T, Matsuura N (1980) Hyperfunctioning thyroid nodules in children. Am J Dis Child 134:961–963
2. Bacon GE, Lowrey GH (1965) Experience with surgical treatment of thyrotoxicosis in children. J Pediatr 67:1–5
3. Barnes HV, Blizzard RM (1977) Antithyroid drug therapy for toxic diffuse goiter (Graves' disease): thirty years' experience in children and adolescents. J Pediatr 91:313–320
4. Boyden SN (1951) Adsorption of proteins on erythrocytes treated with tannic acid and subsequent haemagglutination by antiprotein sera. J Exp Med 93:107–111
5. Bradley III El, Digirolamo M, Tarcan Y (1980) Modified subtotal thyroidectomy in the management of Graves' disease. Surgery 87:623–629
6. Buckingham BA, Costin G, Roe TF, Weitzman JJ, Kogut MD (1981) Hyperthyroidism in children. Am J Dis Child 135:112–117
7. Carey C, Skosey C, Pinnamaneni KM, Barsano CP, DeGroot LJ (1980) Thyroid abnormalities in children of parents who have Graves' disease: possible pre-Graves' disease. Metabolism 29:369–376
8. De Heerk Schnippenkoetter J, Kortmann KB, Beeger R (1984) Postoperativer Verlauf und Taktik der Nachsorge der Hyperthyreose. Chirurg 55:171–173
9. Doniach D (1981) Hashimoto's thyroiditis and primary myxoedema viewed as separate entities (editorial). Eur J Clin Invest 11:245–247
10. Fatourechi V, McConahey WM, Woolner LB (1971) Hyperthyroidism associated with histologic Hashimoto's thyroiditis. May Clin Proc 46:682–689
11. Finke R, Kotulla P, Wenzel B, Bogner V, Meinhold H, Schleusener H (1981) Klinische Bedeutung der Bestimmung von Schilddrüsenstimulierenden Antikörpern. Dtsch Med Wochenschr 106:38–42

12. Freitas JE, Swanson DP, Gross MD, Sisson JC (1979) Iodine-131: optimal therapy for hyperthyroidism in children and adolescents? J Nucl Med 20:847–850
13. Friedman JM, Fialkow PJ (1978) The genetics of Graves' disease. Clin Endocrinol Metab 7:47–65
14. Hothem AL, Thomas CG Jr, Van Wyk JJ (1978) Selection of treatment in the management of thyrotoxicosis in childhood and adolescence. Ann Surg 187:593–598
15. Islam MN, Briones-Urbino R, Bakó Gy, Farid NR (1983) Both TSH and thyroid-stimulating antibody of Graves' disease bind to an M_r 197000 holoreceptor. Endocrinology 113:436–438
16. Junginger T, Kogel H, Winkelmann W (1981) Nachsorge nach operativer Behandlung der Hyperthyreose. In: Rothmund M, Kümmerle F (eds) Fortschritte der endokrinologischen Chirurgie. Thieme, Stuttgart
17. Kálmán K, Fazakas S, Erdei I, Leövey A (1976) Leukocyte migration inhibition in vitro in untreated and methimazole-treated patients with Graves' disease. Acta Med Acad Sci Hung 33:327–332
18. Kálmán K, Erdei I, Sándor P, Fazakas S, Leövey A (1978) Leukocyte migration test for the study of immune reactivity in cases of Graves' disease associated with infiltrative ophthalmopathy. Acta Med Acad Sci Hung 35:94–34
19. Mäenpää J, Kuusi A (1980) Childhood hyperthyroidism. Acta Paediatr Scand 69:137–142
20. McClintock JC, Frawky TF, Holden JHP (1956) Hyperthyroidism in children: observations in 50 treated cases, including an evaluation of endorine factors. J Clin Endocrinol 16:62–85
21. Mühlendahl KE, Helge H (1978) Hyperthyreose im Kindesalter. 2. Klinik und Therapie. Padiatr Prax 20:601–616
22. Perzik SL (1976) The place of total thyroidecotmy in the management of 909 patients with thyroid disease. Am J Surg 132:480–483
23. Roitt I, Doniach D (1969) Immunfluorescent tests for the detection of antibodies. In: WHO manual of autoimmune serology. Geneva
24. Safa AM, Schumacher OP, Rodriguez-Antunez A (1975) Long-arm follow-up results in children and adolescents treated with radioactive iodine (131 I) for hyperthyroidism. N Engl J Med 292:167–171
25. Saxena KM, Crawford JD, Talbot NB (1964) Childhood thyrotoxicosis: a long-term perspective. Br Med J 2:1153–1158
26. Schatz H (1981) Die Bedeutung der Bestimmung von Schilddrüsenantikörpern und der HLA-Typisierung für die Prognose der Hyperthyreose. Med Welt 32:649–652
27. Schatz H, Federlin K (1979) Diagnostik von Immunvergängen bei Schilddrüsenerkrankungen und deren klinische Bedeutung. Med Welt 30:614–618
28. Szabó J, Leövey A (1980) Thyroid antibodies in Graves' disease. An immunofluorescence study. Acta Med Acad Sci Hung 40:91–97
29. Thompson NW, Dunn EL, Freitas JE, Sisson JC, Coran AG, Nishiyama RH (1977) Surgical treatment of thyrotoxicosis in children and adolescents. J Pediatr Surg 12:1009–1017
30. Werner SC (1977) Modification of the classification of the eye changes of Graves' disease: recommendations of the ad hoc committee of the American Thyroid Association. J Clin Endocrinol Metab 44:203–204
31. Wesley JR, Buckingham BA, Gahr JA, Isaacs HJr, Kogut MD, Weitzman JJ (1977) Surgical treatment of hyperthyroidism in children. Surg Gynecol Obstet 145:343–346
32. Young RJ, Sherwood MB, Simpson JG, Nicol AG, Michie W, Becks JS (1976) Histometry of lymphoid infiltrate in the thyroid of primary thyrotoxicosis patients. J Clin Pathol 29:398–402

Late Prognosis
of Childhood and Juvenile Thyroid Carcinomas

G. Balázs[1], G. Lukács[1], G. Csáky[1], P. Boros[2], and I. Ilyés[3]

Summary

The authors report on the biological properties and late prognosis of 16 children and juvenile patients operated on during the past 24 years for thyroid tumour who underwent regular follow-up. The clinical and morphological characteristics of the carcinomas are described, together with the late immune response of the patients undergoing complex treatment. The study is also concerned with the characteristics of the DNA content of the tumorous cell nuclei, the pregnancy success rate of the operated patients and the thyroid function of the children born.

Zusammenfassung

Es wird über die biologischen Eigenheiten und die Spätprognose bei 16 Kindern und Jugendlichen berichtet, die wegen eines Schilddrüsenkarzinoms operiert und regelmäßig nachuntersucht worden waren. Klinische und morphologische Charakteristika der Karzinome sowie die späte Immunantwort der Patienten, die einer komplexen Behandlung unterzogen wurden, werden beschrieben. Die vorliegende Untersuchung befaßt sich ebenfalls mit dem DNS-Gehalt der Tumorzellkerne, der Schwangerschaftserfolgsrate der operierten Patientinnen und der Schilddrüsenfunktion ihrer Kinder.

Résumé

Les auteurs rapportent les particularités biologiques et les prognostics actuels de 16 enfants et adolescents ayant subi une intervention chirurgicale pour tumeur thyroïdienne au cours des 24 dernières années et qui ont été suivis de façon régulière. Ils décrivent les caractéristiques cliniques et morphologiques des carcinomes ainsi que la réponse immunologique récente des patients soumis à un traitement complexe. Cette étude traite aussi des caractéristiques de la teneur en ADN du noyau de la cellule tumorale, de la proportion de grossesses réussies des patientes opérées et de la fonction thyroïdienne de leurs enfants.

We report on the biological properties of thyroid tumours in 16 children and juvenile patients operated on in the past 24 years, thereby providing data for late prognosis.

---

[1]First Department of Surgery,
[2]Third Clinic of Medicine, and
[3]Clinic of Paediatrics, University Medical School of Debrecen, P.O.Box 27, 4012 Debrecen, Hungary.

Progress in Pediatric Surgery, Vol. 26
Gauderer and Angerpointner (Eds.)
© Springer-Verlag Berlin Heidelberg 1991

Material and Method

For the determination of biological property there are no universally accepted parameters in the literature. In our previous papers we considered tumour size, metastasis formation, tendency of the primary tumour to recur, histological structure and survival rate as bases [1, 2]. Recently, in the course of continuous follow-up, the cellular immune response of the patients treated for thyroid carcinoma was determined by parallel application of the leucocyte adhesion and leucocyte migration tests [4]. In addition, the pregnancy success rate of the patients and the general developmental and thyroid functional states of the children born were also considered. More recently, the DNA content of the cell nuclei was measured by cytofluorimetry [11, 12, 13]. Thus, the paper is concerned with four issues:

1. Clinical and morphological characteristics of childhood and juvenile thyroid carcinomas
2. Cellular immune response after complex treatment
3. Characteristic features of the DNA content of the cell nuclei
4. Pregnancy success rate of the patients, thyroid function of the children born

Results

Tumour size is important in view of early diagnosis and radical surgical treatment. It should be noted that of all diagnostic methods we regard as most specific the method of preoperative aspiration and intraoperative imprint cytology. The carcinomas were localized intrathyroidally in all our patients: seven of them belonged to group T1 and nine to T2; thus, none of the tumours adhered to the adjacent cervical organs (Table 1).

Metastasis formation is also characteristic. In ten patients the first clinical symptom was regional lymph node, and in one distant metastasis imitating a miliary pulmonary lesion, which led to the correct diagnosis after preliminary biopsy and histological examination. In the other five cases the indication for surgery was the solitary nodule palpable in the thyroid.

Table 1. pTNM classification of 16 childhood and juvenile thyroid carcinomas, 1962–1978

pT0	pT1	pT2	
–	7	9	= 16
pN0	pN1	pN2	
6	6	4	= 16
pM0	pM1		
15	1		= 16

Table 2. Surgical procedures

Subtotal thyroidectomy	2
Lobectomy + contralateral subtotal resection	11
Total thyroidectomy	3

The histological structure of the tumours is characteristic as well. In addition to 13 cases of papillary carcinoma, there were two follicular tumours and one medullary tumour. The latter belonged to the T1 group and there was still no metastasis. It is notable that the size of the lymph node metastases reached or exceeded the size of the primary tumour.

In view of the recurrence of the primary tumour the decisive factor is the quality of the first surgical procedure and the adjuvant treatment. As seen in Table 2, there were two bilateral subtotal resections and three thyroidectomies, but in the majority of cases preference was given to removal of the tumorous lobe supplemented by contralateral subtotal resection. If there was lymph node metastasis, a modified cervical dissection was performed. Four patients were given X-ray or cobalt irradiation, and one patient ^{131}I supplementary treatment. In addition, all patients have received and continue to receive hormone substitution therapy. With this type of treatment no recurrence of primary tumour has so far occurred. Recurrent regional lymph node metastases were encountered 1.5–2 years postoperatively in four patients. In the course of continuous follow-up no distant metastases have been found; moreover, the only patient with pulmonary metastasis is alive 21 years after the complex treatment and is completely free of complaints [2].

Finally, regarding survival, we can say that 0.5–24 years after the complex treatment all of our patients are alive, and their general state of health corresponds to their ages; their thyroid function, even by hormone analysis, was found to be normal (Fig. 1).

With this knowledge as a basis, the investigation of the cellular immune response of the operated patients seemed instructive, since it can provide further

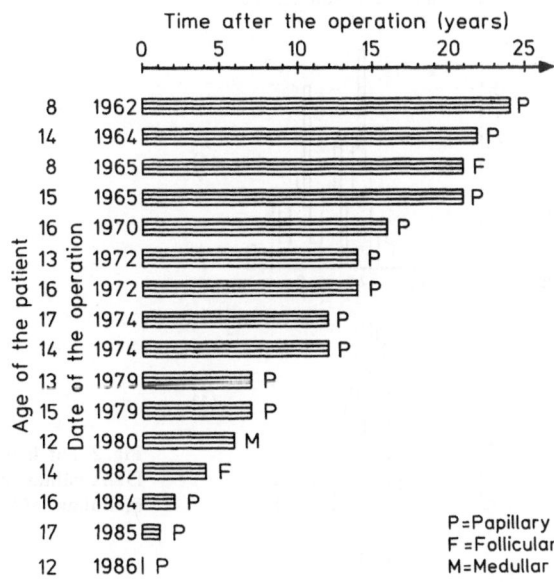

Fig. 1. Survival of the children operated on for thyroid carcinoma 1962–1986

data for the interpretation of special biological properties. It is well known that one form of anti-tumour defence of the human organism is the anti-tumour T-cell-mediated immune response. We have studied the T-cell sensibilization of the patients by parallel application of two methods: leucocyte adhesion inhibition

Table 3. Recognition of tumour-associated antigen by thyroid cancer patients

Time elapsed since the operation	Children No. of positive tests		Adults No. of positive tests	
	LAI	LMT	LAI	LMT
1 year	0/0	0/0	10/14	5/14
1–8 years	2/3	2/3	16/25	11/25
8 years	4/6	2/6	0/ 4	0/ 4
Total	6/9	4/9	26/43	16/43

LAI, Leucocyte adhesion inhibition; LMT, leucocyte migration test

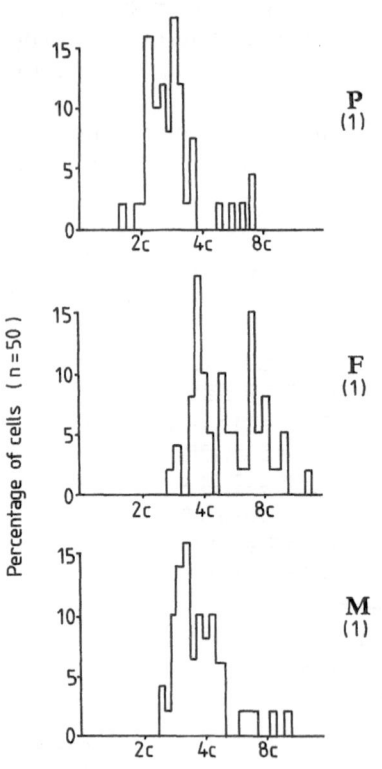

Fig. 2. Nuclear DNA distribution histograms. Modal DNA values of papillary *(P)*, follicular *(F)* and medullary *(M)* thyroid carcinomas are aneuploid

(LAI) and the leucocyte migration test (LMT). The antigen was prepared from papillary thyroid tumour tissue.

According to our results, about half of the patients showed sensibilization against thyroid tumour antigen both with LAI and LMT for a long time − 8–10 years − after the operation (Table 3). Thus, it was not possible to detect factors that would inhibit the sensibilization of T-cells against tumour antigens in the sera of the patients.

Cytochemical tests were performed on the surgically removed tissue in three cases: the DNA content of the cell nuclei was determined by cytofluorimetry. Whereas the relative DNA content of normal thyroid epithelial cells is identical with the diploid (2c) value, in all forms of malignant tumours a considerable elevation is encountered with aneuploid cell distribution (Fig. 2). Similar conclusions have been drawn by other authors [3, 6].

At different times after the complex treatment, three of our patients became pregnant. After uneventful pregnancies, these patients delivered five live-born mature neonates, with weights above 3000 g (Table 4). During and after their pregnancies the mothers were given substitution therapy. The thyroid state of the neonates and small children was normal. No hypothyroidism or factitial hyperthyroidism has so far occurred.

The somatic development of the children born proved to be normal, their percentual values for weight and length fell within the normal range. On physical

Table 4. Pregnancies after operations

Case	Date of		Histology	Birth weight (g)
	Operation	Birth		
1	1962	1973	Papillary	3700
		1976		3300
2	1965	1973	Papillary	3000
		1975		3100
3	1974	1976	Papillary	3200

Table 5. Thyroid function of the children

	T_3U	T_4-RIA (nmol)	FT_4I [a]	TSH (mU/l)
1	1.05	113.3	118.9	2.5
2	1.03	132.6	136.5	2.3
3	1.00	118.4	118.4	2.2
4	0.93	110.7	103.0	4.1
5	0.96	115.8	111.2	3.4
Mean ± SD	0.99 ± 0.05	118.2 ± 8.7	117.6 ± 12.4	2.9 ± 0.8

[a] $FT_4I = T_3U \times T_4$-RIA

examination no case of goitre was found in any of them. To evaluate their thyroid function the T_3U test was performed; the T_4 and TSH concentrations were determined with the RIA method, and from the T_3U and T_4-RIA values the so-called free T_4 index (FT_4I) was calculated (Table 5). Both the individual and average values fell within the normal range. The titres of thyroglobulin and microsomal antibodies were also determined: titres $1:16$ or higher were not encountered.

Discussion

Few reports have so far been published on the biological properties and long follow-up of childhood thyroid carcinomas [5, 7–10]. Interestingly, anaplastic cancer hardly occurs at this age, and medullary carcinoma is also considered rare [14]. In our material of 400 patients with thyroid carcinoma, the proportion of anaplastic tumours is 20%. No such tumour has been seen among the cases of childhood carcinoma. The favourable prognosis of childhood thyroid carcinomas can be attributed mainly to slow tumour growth, intrathyroidal localization, its mostly papillary structure, the rarity of recurrence of primary tumour and the benign metastases. These patients do not show general tumorous symptoms. Their development corresponds to that of their age group; with regard to work capacity they are citizens of full value. This is why, together with Röhrer [15], we consider the less radical surgical solution justified.

It is worthy of note that the patients who have undergone complex treatment show, for a long time after the operation, sensibilization against thyroid tumour antigen. Therefore, it is recommended that the immunological tests be repeated at certain intervals – every 0.5–1 year – since it can be assumed that decrease in the reactivity of the T-cells may predict the progress of the tumour.

The treated and regularly followed up patient can, with full responsibility and a fair prognosis, take on the task of founding a family. The general development of the children born and their thyroid function do not seem to be influenced by the earlier disease of the mother.

References

1. Balázs Gy, Bánfi J, Péter F (1974) Biologische Eigenschaften des kindlichen und juvenilen Schilddrüsenkrebses. Z Kinderchir 14:366–373
2. Balázs Gy, Csáky G, Lukács G, Bánfi J, Péter F, Krajczár G (1979) Biologische Eigenschaften des kindlichen und juvenilen Schilddrüsenkrebses. Erfahrungen von 17 Jahren bei 11 Patienten. Z Kinderchir 28:225–232
3. Bengtsson A, Malmaeus J, Grimelius L, Johansson H, Pontén J, Rastad J, Akerström G (1984) Measurement of nuclear DNA content in thyroid diagnosis. World J Surg 8:481–486
4. Boros P, Csáky, G, Balázs Gy, Szegedi Gy (1986) Zellularimmunologische Untersuchungen beim kindlichen und juvenilen Schilddrüsenkrebs. Zentralbl Chir 111:1179–1182
5. Bretzel RG, Schatz M (1985) Prognostische Faktoren beim Schilddrüsenkarzinom. Zentralbl Chir 110:1304–1314

6. Cohn K, Bäckdahl M, Forsslund G, Auer G, Lundell G, Löwhagen T, Tallroth E, Willems JS (1984) Prognostic value of nuclear DNA content in papillary thyroid cancer. World J Surg 8:474–480

7. Gottschild D, Zinner G, Langbein Th, Neumann G, Wünsche A, Schneider G (1986) Zur Therapie des Schilddrüsenkarzinoms im Kindes- und Jugendalter aus radiologischer Sicht. Radiobiol Radiother (Berl) 27:709–720

8. Jääskeläinen MK, Lamberg BA (1985) Differentiated thyroid carcinoma in children. In: Jaffiol C, Milhaud G (eds) Thyroid carcinoma. Elsevier, Amsterdam, pp 357–358

9. Joppich I, Röhrer HD, Hecker WCh, Kuorr D, Daum R (1980) Besonderheiten des Schilddrüsenkarzinoms im Kindesalter. Klin Padiatr 192:436–439

10. Keminger K (1983) Die Lebenserwartung bei Schilddrüsenkarzinom in der Jugend. Zentralbl Chir 108:513–520

11. Lukács GL, Balázs Gy, Zs.-Nagy I (1979) Cytofluorimetric measurements on the DNA contents of tumor cells in human thyroid gland. J Cancer Res Clin Oncol 95:265–271

12. Lukács GL, Mikó T, Fábián E, Zs.-Nagy I, Csáky G, Balázs Gy (1983) The validity of some morphological methods in the diagnosis of thyroid malignancy. Acta Chir Scand 149:759–766

13. Lukács GL, Zs.-Nagy I, Lustyik Gy, Balázs Gy (1983) Microfluorometric and X-ray microanalytic studies on the DNA content and $Na^+:K^+$ ratios of the cell nuclei in various types of thyroid tumors. J Cancer Res Clin Oncol 105:280–284

14. Meybier H, Schmidt-Gayk H, Schutze U (1982) Die C-Zell-Tumoren der Schilddrüse im Kindesalter. Z Kinderchir 36:30–33

15. Röhrer HD (1983) Zugänge und Radikalität bei der chirurgischen Behandlung des Schilddrüsen-Carcinoms. Langenbecks Arch Chir 359:1–4

Parathyroid Surgery in Children

A.J. Ross, III

Summary

Parathyroid surgery in children is uncommon. Spontaneously occurring cases of hyperparathyroidism are almost always due to single-gland disease; however, on exploration all four parathyroid glands should be identified. Most of the other instances in which the surgeon needs to perform a parathyroidectomy on an infant or a child will be situations were multiple-gland disease is the rule rather than the exception. Therefore, the surgeon must have in his mind a well developed logical approach to the management of children with parathyroid disorders on the basis of multiple glandular disease. We believe that the technique of parathyroid autotransplantation very satisfactorily addresses the surgical needs of children with familial hyperparathyroid states, including the multiple endocrine neoplasias. We believe that it is mandatory treatment in patients presenting with neonatal primary hyperparathyroidism and is also the procedure of choice in children with secondary and tertiary hyperparathyroidism. The workup and diagnosis of parathyroid disorders should be familiar to the surgeon who undertakes neck exploration on children, and the entity of familial hypocalciuric hypercalcemia should be looked for, as these patients have a strong likelihood of not benefiting from parathyroidectomy.

Zusammenfassung

Operationen der Nebenschilddrüse bei Kindern sind selten. Spontan auftretende Fälle von Hyperparathyreoidismus beruhen fast immer auf der Erkrankung einer einzelnen Drüse. Es sollten jedoch bei der Operation alle 4 Nebenschilddrüsenkörperchen identifiziert werden. Bei den meisten anderen Fällen, wo der Chirurg bei Säuglingen oder Kindern eine Parathyroidektomie durchführen muß, liegt in der Regel eine Erkrankung mehrerer Drüsen anstatt nur einer vor. Daher muß der Chirurg ein klares Konzept der Behandlung von Kindern mit Erkrankungen mehrerer Nebenschilddrüsenkörperchen haben. Es wird die Auffassung vertreten, daß die Technik der Nebenschilddrüsenautotransplantation den chirurgischen Erfordernissen bei Kindern mit familiärem Hyperparathyreoidismus inklusive der multiplen endokrinen Neoplasien entspricht. Diese Technik ist ebenfalls die Methode der Wahl bei Patienten mit neonatalem Hyperparathyreoidismus sowie bei Kindern mit sekundärem und tertiärem Hyperparathyreoidismus. Der Chirurg, der Explorationen der Halsregion vornimmt, sollte mit der Diagnostik von Nebenschilddrüsenerkrankungen vertraut sein. Es soll auf das Krankheitsbild der familiären hypokalziurischen Hyperkalziämie geachtet werden, da diese Patienten höchstwahrscheinlich von einer Parathyroidektomie nicht profitieren werden.

Assistant Professor of Surgery, University of Pennsylvania School of Medicine and Attending Surgeon, The Children's Hospital of Philadelphia, 34th Street and Civic Center Boulevard, Philadelphia, PA 19104, USA.

Progress in Pediatric Surgery, Vol. 26
Gauderer and Angerpointner (Eds.)
© Springer-Verlag Berlin Heidelberg 1991

Résumé

L'ablation chirurgicale des glandes parathyroïdes chez les enfants est rare. Les cas d'hyperpara-thyroïdie survenue spontanément sont presque toujours dus à une affection d'une seule glande; il faudra malgré tout toujours vérifier les quatre glandes. Dans la plupart des cas pout lesquels une parathyroïdectomie s'impose, il y a affection multiple des glandes. Il faut donc que le chir-urgien ait mis en place un plan thérapeutique logique pour le traitement des enfants présentant des troubles parathyroïdien dus à des affections glandulaires multiples. A notre avis, la technique d'autotransplantation parathyroïdienne répond parfaitement aux besoins des enfants de familles où les cas d'hyperparathyroïdie sont fréquents, y compris les néoplasies endocrines multiples. Pour nons ce traitement s'impose absolument dans le cas de patients présentant une hyperpara-thyroïdie néonatale primaire et reste aussi le traitement de choix des hyperparathyroïdies secon-daires et tertiaires. Le chirurgien se doit de connaître parfaitement la méthode de diagnostic des troubles parathyroïdiens quand il examine le cou des enfants et de prendre en considération une possibilité d'hypercalcémie hypocalciurique familiale qui risquerait fort de compromettre les résultats de la parathyroïdectomie.

Introduction

The advent of routine screening utilizing multichannel biochemical analyzers has increased detection of parathyroid disorders in the adult population; however, the incidence of spontaneously occurring parathyroid disease in children remains quite low. This not withstanding, the pediatric surgeon is occasionally asked to participate in the management of a child with a parathyroid disorder. In addition to spontaneous disease, certain populations of children have an increased risk for the presence of a disorder of the parathyroid glands. Often it is predictable as to whether there is single or multiple gland disease. This chapter will review the types of hyperparathyroidism encountered in children and outline the appropriate management for such childen.

Pathophysiology

Parathyroid hormone is an 84-amino-acid single-chain polypeptide that is synthe-sized, stored in, and released from the parathyroid glands. Once secreted, the hormone is cleaved into amino (N) terminal and carboxy (C) terminal fragments. The N-terminal fragment is biochemically active and rapidly metabolized, whereas the C-terminal fragment is more stable and serves as a good serum mark-er for assay purposes. Careful autopsy studies have shown than in more than 90% of cases four parathyroid glands are present, and the syndrome of hyper-parathyroidism is caused by overactivity of either a single gland or multiple glands [1, 2].

The primary function of parathyroid hormone is to control calcium concentra-tion within the extracellular fluid, and the mechanism of action of the hormone is exerted at the renal level by stimulating the rate of reabsorption of calcium from the glomerular filtrate, and in bone by influencing the rate of calcium reabsorption from the skeleton. Additionally, through interaction with vitamin D and its metabolites, an indirect effect of parathyroid hormone exists at the gut level via vitamin D-mediated absorption of calcium. Parathyroid hormone also influences the concentration of phosphate in the extracellular fluid via its phosphaturic action upon the kidney.

In primary states of hyperparathyroidism, regardless of whether one or multiple glands are involved, the physical and biochemical findings are explained by idiopathic glandular overactivity. This differs from states of secondary hyperparathyroidism, where the hypersecretion of parathyroid hormone is a compensatory reaction following the chronic tendency toward hypocalcemia due to problems such as the impaired formation of 1,25 dihydroxy vitamin D, so it is important to know whether the specific type of parathyroid disorder is primary or secondary when dealing with any child with hyperparathyroidism and whether it is due to the overactivity of a single or multiple glands.

Diagnosis

The hallmarks of the diagnosis of primary hyperparathyroidism are hypercalcemia, hypophosphatemia, and an elevated parathyroid hormone level. It is known that the parathyroid hormone-enhanced renal loss of phosphate and bicarbonate creates a compensatory retention of chloride in patients with primary hyperparathyroidism; Palmer et al. have suggested that an elevated chloride phosphate (Cl/P) ratio is good means of discriminating hyperparathyroidism from other causes of hypercalcemia and we, too, have found it helpful [3, 4]. A 24-h urine determination for calcium with the patient on a controlled diet should be performed on any child undergoing consideration for primary hyperparathyroidism, as low levels of urinary calcium excretion in the presence of hypercalcemia may suggest the presence of familial hypocalciuric hypercalcemia – an important diagnosis, since these children may not benefit from parathyroidectomy. An array of parathyroid hormone assays are available, and they have been designed to look at both the intact molecule and its fragments. Assays directed toward the C-terminal fragment should be diagnostic of primary hyperparathyroidism in most instances. The more sophisticated assay analyses should be performed only when the diagnosis is in question or problematic.

Radiographic means of aiding in the diagnosis of primary hyperparathyroidism have traditionally been helpful only in advanced cases where subperiosteal resorption has been detectable either in the finger tips or at the acromioclavicular articulations. Recently, other imaging techniques have been utilized preoperatively to localize functioning parathyroid adenomas. These include real-time ultrasound, dual isotope scintigraphy, and high-resolution MR imaging [5–7]. In experienced hands each of these techniques seems to have high sensitivity, and at the current time their utility seems to be greatest in the preoperative localization of an adenoma in the child in whom the diagnosis of primary hyperparathyroidism cannot otherwise be confirmed, or in the patient who has undergone a prior neck exploration. The value of their application in the routine evaluation of the child with primary hyperparathyroidism has yet to be established.

Specific aids in the diagnosis of many of the individual parathyroid syndromes, as well as the differential diagnosis, are covered in the discussions of these entities.

Clinical Disorders

Spontaneous Primary Hyperparathyroidism

The most common spontaneous cause of primary hyperparathyroidism in children is a single adenoma. This entity is relatively rare; the recent reviews of Girard and Allo [8, 9] detail the fact that there are slightly more than 100 cases reported in the world literature to date. These and other series suggest that the incidence is somewhat higher in males than in females and that its onset is rare before the age of 10 years. Nonspecific symptoms such as weakness, malaise, and fatigue are commonplace, as are anorexia and irritability. Rappaport suggests that the incidences of bone disease and renal involvement are higher in children than in adults, presumably due to the high average duration of disease in children prior to its recognition [10].

Evaluation of hypercalcemia in the patient with spontaneously occurring hyperparathyroidism follows the guidelines outlined earlier. Specific diagnoses such as sarcoidosis, osteoporosis due to prolonged bed rest, milk-alkali syndrome, and malignancy all must be ruled out, as must the possibility that the hypercalcemia is caused by medication such as a thiazide diuretic. Furthermore, thought should be given to the presence of familial hypocalciuric hypercalcemia, discussed in more detail later.

The etiology of spontaneously occurring hyperparathyroidism in children remains uncertain, as it does in adults. Recently, Nishiyama et al. suggested a possible relationship between sporadic parathyroid adenomas and prior head and neck radiation [11]. This group has seen an increasing number of patients with parathyroid adenomas who have previously had 131-iodine thyroid ablation for Grave's disease. It is yet to be determined whether more parathyroid adenomas are detected in patients who have undergone ^{131}I treatment during childhood, adolescence or early adulthood, but since the therapy is being employed with increasing frequency, the answer should be clear within this decade.

Once the diagnosis is secured, the patients are treated by exploratory neck surgery. There seems to be little place, if any, for medical management of primary hyperparathyroidism, especially in this population of children who are otherwise healthy. We utilize the technique of neck exploration described by Wells et al. [4], where by exposure is gained through a transverse collar incision and the strap muscles are retracted rather than divided. In every instance all four parathyroid glands are identified, as are both recurrent laryngeal nerves. Nonabsorable suture tags are placed directly adjacent to each of the normal glands. Despite the fact that in this population virtually all patients will have a single enlarged gland, we believe that it is important to have identified all four glands before removing the adenoma, and, of course, frozen section confirmation is mandatory. The individual surgeon's experience and expertise dictate whether biopsies should be obtained of the "normal" glands; however, at the very least, their gross identification is mandatory.

Postoperatively, these patients may have a precipitous fall in their serum calcium, so serum calcium levels should be monitored until they are found to have become stable. It is our preference not to treat this relative hypocalcemia unless the patient becomes specifically symptomatic.

Familial Hyperparathyroidism

In 1936, Goldman and Smith first suggested that primary hyperparathyroidism could be inherited on the basis of their experience with its occurrence in two siblings [12]. Primary hyperparathyroidism may occur on a genetic basis either as an isolated disorder or coincident with other endocrinopathies. The most essential feature for the surgeon to bear in mind is that with virtually all of these disorders the parathyroid pathology is hyperplasia of multiple glands. Familial hyperparathyroidism on the basis of a single adenoma is exceedingly rare, so neck exploration and surgical management in these patients should be designed according to the individual surgeon's approach and training for the management of multiple gland disease [13].

Multiple endocrine adenomatosis types I and II (also known as the multiple endocrine neoplasias) are inherited in an autosomal dominant fashion and are often associated with parathyroid hyperplasia. *Multiple endocrine adenomatosis type I* is the more common of these two syndromes, and hyperparathyroidism is frequently the first lesion to present in this endocrinopathy [14]. Also involved in this constellation of abnormal endocrine organs are the pituitary gland, which may demonstrate an adenoma or hyperfunction, and the pancreas, which often contains a gastrin-secreting tumor producing the Zollinger-Ellison syndrome. The thyroid and adrenal glands may also be involved to a lesser extent with adenomas. It is rare for symptoms of any sort to present in MEA type I within the first decade of life, and the patient is frequently well into adulthood before symptoms or biochemical disturbances are noted. Whereas hypercalcemia may be the first detectable stigma of this syndrome in screened patients, the first clinical symptoms have tended to be due to peptic ulcer disease [15]. In view of the fact that more than 90% of patients with this syndrome will have hyperparathyroidism, initial screening efforts should be directed toward this finding. It is uncommon for a child to manifest hypercalcemia before adolescence, so screening should be started at about the age of 10 years. *Multiple endocrine adenomatosis type II* is also genetically determined in an autosomal dominant fashion. The most common lesion seen in this endocrinopathy is medullary carcinoma of the thyroid, present in virtually 100% of patients; however, pheochromocytoma (40%) and hyperparathyroidism (60%) occur with great frequency as well [16]. As in MEA type I, the clinical manifestations of this disorder are not generally seen within the first decade of life. On the other hand, since the diagnosis of this syndrome may often be made in a precancerous state (C-cell hyperplasia) utilizing calcitonin provocative studies, we and others feel that yearly screening should be undertaken beginning in childhood [17]. Should a member of an MEA type II kindred be uncovered and require surgery, the presence of a coincident pheochromocytoma must be ruled out prior to the induction of a general anesthetic. Interestingly, the small percentage of patients who are found to have MEA type II B rarely develop hyperparathyroidism, so management of multiple gland parathyroid disease is not an issue in these patients.

Solitary autosomal dominant hyperparathyroidism is the only endocrine disorder in some kindreds. When found as an isolated trait in patients who are also hypercalciuric, treatment considerations are the same as in the other familial endocrinopathies; as a rule, one finds multiglandular disease. A critical distinction must be made between this entity and another autosomal dominant hypercalcemic disorder; *familial hypocalciuric hypercalcemia* (FHH). This syndrome, first introduced by Foley et al. in 1972, has as its components (a) hypercalcemia without other endocrine features of multiple endocrine neoplasia type I or type II; (b) hypercalcemia with relative hypocalciuria; (c) hypercalcemia before age 10; and (d) the inability to maintain normocalcemia after parathyroidectomy [18]. In many instances the familial benign hypocalciuric hypercalcemic situation is asymptomatic and is detected serendipitously or is found as a result of family studies. Researchers who have recently investigated this disease have all urged evaluation for the presence of this entity in any patient suspected of having hyperparathyroidism [19–22]. This is due to the fact that, with one exception, the hypercalcemia is often not corrected with parathyroidectomy and, in view of the benign course of FHH, parathyroidectomy is usually not necessary. The exception to this case is the rare infant who is born with signs and symptoms of congenital hyperparathyroidism presenting as symptomatic hypercalcemia at birth. Neonatal hyperparathyroidism also has an autosomal recessive basis and this is discussed separately in the section on neonatal hyperparathyroidism.

The surgical management of patients with each of these types of familial hyperparathyroidism reflects, in a large part, the individual surgeon's approach to the management of multiple parathyroid gland disease, as virtually all of these patients have the propensity to, if not the existence of, multiply involved parathyroid glands. Whereas it seems reasonable in sporadic parathyroid hyperfunction to identify all four parathyroid glands and to remove only those glands proven on biopsy to be abnormal, the high incidence of chief cell hyperplasia involving all four parathyroid glands in familial hyperparathyroidism disorders dictates that the individual surgeon's personal approach toward four-gland disease always be employed. This is an important consideration because, grossly, there may be a distinct variation in the size of the parathyroid glands, such that some are clearly enlarged whereas others may appear to be normal. Furthermore, all glands must be identified and biopsied, as it is not at all uncommon for a "normal" sized gland to have hyperplastic changes clearly demonstrable upon microscopic examination.

Many have employed and utilized the technique of 3 ½-gland parathyroidectomy in the management of four-gland disease. This spares a total of 30–50 mg of parathyroid tissue. Although success has been reported with this technique, there are high rates of complications of recurrent or persistent hyperparathyroidism in this population. Indeed, as many as 30%–50% of these patients have required neck reexploration. Such procedures are technically more difficult than are initial neck explorations and are associated with a far greater risk of recurrent laryngeal nerve damage as well as prolonged permanent hypoparathyroidism [23–26]. These concerns led to the introduction, in 1976, of the application of parathyroid autotransplantation for these patients [27]. This technique was developed as a more effective means of dealing with patients with four-gland disease, which is so often present in this population. Following identification and removal of all four glands, one is divided into slivers of 1–2 mm which are implanted into the volar aspect of the nondominant forearm marked with individual nonabsorbable sutures. Postoperatively, once the patient is symptomatically hypocalcemic, calcium and vitamin D are administered until graft function occurs – usually in 10–21 days [4, 28]. The success of the technique has been well documented and can be successfully accomplished in almost all patients with no appreciable incidence of late graft failure. Recurrence of hypercalcemia in familial hyperparathyroid patients is a difficult problem and occurs with this technique, too, but it is far more safely and easily managed with graft removal from the forearm than with neck reexploration, which is historically both hazardous and unsuccessful [29]. Our approach to patients with MEA type II who have no biochemical evidence of hyperparathyroidism, and in patients with MEA type IIB, has been that of total thyroidectomy for their medullary carcinoma with preservation of the parathyroid glands. We feel that if a total thyroidectomy cannot be performed without jeopardizing the blood supply to the parathyroids, as is so often the case, the parathyroids should be transplanted into the sternocleidomastoid muscle, where they will function well. It is more important to accomplish the complete thyroidectomy than it is to preserve the blood supply to the parathyroids in this disorder, and the decision to transplant into the sternocleidomastoid muscle should be made. On the basis of the fact that MEA type IIA patients seem to have less "severe" parathyroid disease with a lower likelihood of recurrence, it has been recommended that consideration be given to excision of the enlarged parathyroid glands only, and that the patient not undergo an empiric 3 ½-gland parathyroidectomy or parathyroid autotransplant. It must be emphasized that, in our view, there must be unequivocal histologic proof of normal parathyroid gland anatomy before any consideration is given to employing this approach. As always, individual consideration of each patient and each surgeon's training and expertise are of paramount importance when designing the appropriate operative procedure for any of these patients.

Primary Hyperparathyroidism in Infancy

This is a rare and interesting disorder; at the time of our recent review, we found 29 cases reported in the world literature [30]. Neonatal primary hyperparathyroidism uniformly presents within the first 3 months of life, usually at or shortly following birth. The histologic finding in 100% of afflicted neonates is hyperplasia of all four parathyroid glands. The predominant symptoms include hypotonicity, respiratory distress, failure to thrive, constipation, anorexia, irritability, lethargy, and polyuria. These babies often have impressive roentgenograms demonstrating pathologic fractures as well as subperiosteal bone resorption and osteoporosis. Although Goldman and Smith, in 1936, first recognized that hyperparathyroidism could be familial, it was not proven until 1964, when Hillman et al. described neonatal primary hyperparathyroidism in two siblings born to first-cousin parents [12, 31]. Since that time, it has become apparent that this phenotpye can be inherited in an autosomal recessive fashion, and in our review we found that approximately half of the affected infants reported had a familial tendency toward hyperparathyroidism.

The differential diagnosis of neonatal hyperparathyroidism includes such disorders as neonatal hyperparathyroidism associated with maternal hypoparathyroidism, idiopathic infantile hypercalcemia, subcutaneous fat necrosis, and blue diaper syndrome [32–35]. Additionally, cases of hypercalcemia due to mesoblastic nephroma have also been reported; the pathogenesis of the hypercalcemia in these infants was felt to be prostaglandin E-related [36]. Whereas hypercalcemia has frequently been reported as a sequela of cancer in adults, this is one of the few instances where hypercalcemia (other than due to bone metastases) occurs in infants with a malignancy. The serum calcium returns to normal following management of the mesoblastic nephroma.

Infants with neonatal primary hyperparathyroidism often seem to display a clinical and biochemical phenotype similar to those with the FHH syndrome. Their disease, however, is an exception to the usual benign nature of FHH which is typically detected later in life, as afflicted babies are usually critically ill.

As medical management of neonatal primary hyperparathyroidism resulted in near certain death, the severe nature of the illness in infants presenting with this condition led to the recommendation for urgent parathyroidectomy. Subtotal 3 ½-gland parathyroidectomy was initially performed, but this, too, was found to be unacceptable due to the almost uniform recurrence of disease. Whereas total parathyroidectomy was later employed, it led to the need for lifelong replacement of calcium and vitamin D, which is a difficult management problem. Due to a basic dissatisfaction with these therapeutic options, we and two other groups have utilized total parathyroidectomy with parathyroid autotransplantation when confronted with neonates with this disorder [30, 37, 38]. All of the children have responded successfully to this approach and have done well, leading us to recommend total parathyroidectomy with parathyroid autotransplantation for the rare neonate with primary hyperparathyroidism. A neonate of an FHH kindred is reported for whom the illness was substantially less devastating than for most infants who have presented with neonatal hyperparathyroidism. In view of the child's family history and his controllable disease, this child was managed, successfully, in an expectant nonsurgical fashion. It would seem that for such infants with a family history of FHH the initial therapy could be conservative if the baby's critical cardiorespiratory functions and development are not compromised by the hypercalcemia [39].

Secondary Hyperparathyroidism

A compensatory state of hypersecretion of parathyroid hormone is termed secondary hyperparathyroidism, and this tends to occur in any clinical condition in which there is a tendency toward hypocalcemia. The prolonged survival of patients with renal insufficiency utilizing hemodialysis is perhaps the best example of this phenomenon, but the disorder is not limited to this population. Secondary hyperparathyroidism can present in certain instances of rickets or osteomalacia, as well as in intestinal malabsorption syndromes. Typically, all of these states manifest normal-to-low serum calcium levels, with the most marked manifestation of the secondary hyperparathyroidism in the skeletal system. In the secondary hyperparathyroidism of chronic renal failure, surgical intervention is often beneficial, whereas in the other entities medical management is generally successful.

Severe skeletal involvement in the patient with renal failure is termed renal osteodystrophy. A small percentage of these patients are refractory to conservative therapy directed toward reducing phosphorus absorption and using vitamin D to increase calcium absorption. In such patients, the development of skeletal fractures, intractable pruritus, or metastatic calcification of the vascular system or soft tissues is an indication for parathyroidectomy.

Whereas some clinicians have recommended total parathyroidectomy with use of oral vitamin D and calcium replacement therapy in this population of patients, others have suggested that a subtotal (3½-gland) parathyroidectomy be performed. Our belief, however, is that this represents another clinical indication for the use of parathyroid autotransplantation. Again, avoided are the difficult management problems of lifelong vitamin D and calcium replacement in the aparathyroid patient, as well as the hazard of neck reexploration in patients with persistent or recurring hyperparathyroidism. Again, with autotransplantation of parathyroid tissue to the forearm, a portion of the autograft could be excised should graft-dependent hyperfunction ultimately be encountered. It is our belief that the performance of parathyroid autotransplantation and resolution of the renal osteodystrophy ultimately makes the patient a better candidate for renal transplantation [28].

Kinder and Rasmussen have recently shown that parathyroid autotransplantation is of benefit in selected patients with secondary hyperparathyroidism due to familial hypophosphatemic rickets or pseudohypoparathyroidism. In their patients the metabolic bone disease responded nicely to this therapeutic intervention [40].

Tertiary Hyperparathyroidism

There is an interesting population of patients with hyperparathyroidism secondary to chronic renal failure who, after kidney transplantation and resumption of "normal" renal function, develop signs and symptoms of hypercalcemia due to the continued overproduction of parathyroid hormone by the four hyperplastic parathyroid glands. This is termed tertiary hyperparathyroidism. Although actual damage to the transplanted kidney by the hypercalcemia is not well documented, the patients may have all of the constitutional and psychomotor disturbances so often noted in primary hyperparathyroidism. As all four glands are, by definition, enlarged in this situation, we recommend that parathyroid autotransplantation be performed in this clinical condition as well.

Parathyroid Allotransplantation

Of all indications for parathyroid surgery in children, those for parathyroid allotransplantation are the most uncommon. Some years ago it was believed that parathyroid was an immunologically privileged tissue. This hypothesis was never conclusively demonstrated and this has not been our experience clinically; we have reported on a patient who had the rapid concurrent rejection of both his renal and parathyroid allotransplants after 30 months of function [41]. Currently, we feel that, at least in man, parathyroid tissue is not privileged immunologically, and it seems that the pharmacologic immunosupression which would be required for successful allotransplantation likely presents a potentially greater risk of morbidity than the vitamin D and oral calcium replacement therapy required. On the other hand, in the rarely encountered situation where hypoparathyroidism is refractory to pharmacologic management, consideration should be given to parathyroid allotransplantation in the appropriately immunosuppressed host utilizing a "match" of maximal tissue histocompatibility. For patients with DeGeorge's syndrome, a disease characterized by absence of the pharyngeal pouch derivatives (parathyroid and thymus), allotransplantation of the parathyroid glands could theoretically be accomplished without immunosuppression. The other coincident findings in such patients − for example, severe cardiac disease − have not enabled this hypothesis to be well tested in man.

References

1. Alveryd A (1968) Parathyroid glands in thyroid surgery. Acta Chir Scand [Suppl]389:1–120
2. Akerstrom G, Malmaers J, Bergstrom R (1984) Surgical anatomy of human parathyroid glands. Surgery 95:14–21
3. Palmer FJ, Nelson JC, Bacchus H (1974) The chloride-phosphate ratio in hypercalcemia. Ann Intern Med 80:200–204
4. Wells SA Jr, Leight GS, Ross AJ III (1980) Primary hyperparathyroidism. In: Ravitch MM, Steichen FM (eds) Current problems in surgery, vol 17. Yearbook Medical, Chicago, pp 397–464

5. Allen DB, Friedman AL, Hendricks SA (1986) Asymptomatic primary hyperparathyroidism in children − newer methods of preoperative diagnosis. Am J Dis Child 140:819–821
6. Gordon L, Carr D (1986) Preoperative localization of parathyroid adenomas using thalium-technetium subtraction scintigraphy. South Med J 79:1337–1338
7. Spritzer CE, Gefter WB, Hamilton R, Greenberg BM, Axel L, Kressel HY (1987) Abnormal parathyroid glands: high-resolution MR imaging. Radiology 162:487–491
8. Allo M, Thompson NW, Nishiyama R (1982) Primary hyperparathyroidism in children, adolescents and young adults. World J Surg 6:771–776
9. Girard RM, Belanger A, Hazel B (1982) Primary hyperparathyroidism in children. Can J Surg 25:11–16
10. Rapaport D, Ziv Y, Rubin M, Huminer D, Dintsman M (1986) Primary hyperparathyroidism in children. J Pediatr Surg 21:395–397
11. Nishiyama RH, Farhi D, Thompson NW (1979) Radiation exposure and the simultaneous occurrence of primary hyperparathyroidism and thyroid nodules. Surg Clin North Am 59:65–75
12. Goldman L, Smith FS (1936) Hyperparathyroidism in siblings. Ann Surg 104:971–981
13. Allo M, Thompson NW (1982) Familial hyperparathyroidism caused by solitary adenomas. Surgery 92:486–490
14. Benson L, Ljunghall S, Akerstrom G, Oberg K (1987) Hyperparathyroidism presenting as the first lesion in multiple endocrine neoplasia type I. Am J Med 82:731–737
15. Ballard HS, Frame B, Hartsock RJ (1964) Familial multiple endocrine adenoma-peptic ulcer complex. Medicine 43:481–516
16. Wells SA Jr, Baylin SB (1986) The multiple endocrine neoplasias. In: Sabiston DC (ed) Textbook of surgery. Saunders, Philadelphia, pp 611–619
17. Graham SM, Genel M, Touloukian RJ, Barwick KW, Gertner JM, Torony C (1987) Provocative testing for occult medullary carcinoma of the thyroid: findings in seven children with multiple endocrine neoplasia type II-A. J Pediatr Surg 22:501–503
18. Foley TP Jr, Harrison HC, Arnaud CD, et al (1972) Familial benign hypercalcemia. J Pediatr 81:1060–1067
19. Marx SJ, Attie MF, Spiegel AM, Levine MA, Lasker RD, Fox M (1982) An association between neonatal severe primary hyperparathyroidism and familial hypocalciuric hypercalcemia. N Engl J Med 306:257–264
20. Marx SJ, Fraser D, Rapoport A (1985) Familial hypocalciuric hypercalcemia − mild expression of the gene in heterozygotes and severe expression in homozygotes. Am J Med 78:15–22
21. Lyons TJ, Crookes PF, Postlethwaite W, Sheridan B, Brown RC, Atkinson AB (1986) Familial hypocalciuric hypercalcemia as a differential diagnosis of hyperparathyroidism: studies in a large kindred and a review of the surgical experience in the condition. Br J Surg 73:188–192
22. Law WM, Heath H III (1985) Familial benign hypercalcemia (hypocalciuric hypercalcemia). Ann Intern Med 102:511–519
23. Castleman B, Cope O (1951) Primary parathyroid hyperplasia. Bull Hosp Jt Dis 12:368–378
24. Castleman B, Schantz A, Roth SI (1976) Parathyroid hyperplasia in primary hyperparathyroidism. Cancer 38:1668–1675
25. Edis AJ, Heerden JA van, Scholz DA (1979) Results of subtotal parathyroidectomy for primary chief cell hyperplasia. Surgery 86:462–469
26. Heerden JA van, Kent RB, Sizemore GW, Grant CS, Remine WH (1983) Primary hyperparathyroidism in patients with multiple endocrine neoplasia syndromes. Arch Surg 118:533–536
27. Wells SA Jr, Ellis GJ, Gunnells JC, et al (1976) Parathyroid autotransplantation in primary parathyroid hyperplasia. N Engl J Med 295:57–62
28. Wells SA Jr, Ross AJ III, Dale JK, et al (1979) Transplantation of the parathyroid glands: current status. Surg Clin North Am 59:167–177
29. Wells SA Jr, Farndon JR, Dale JK (1980) Long-term evaluation of patients with primary parathyroid hyperplasia managed by total parathyroidectomy and heterotopic autotransplantation. Ann Surg 192:451–458

30. Ross AJ III, Cooper A, Attie MF, Bishop HC (1986) Primary hyperparathyroidism in infancy. J Pediatr Surg 21:493–499
31. Hillman DA, Scriver CR, Pedvis S, et al (1964) Neonatal familial primary hyperparathyroidism. N Engl J Med 270:483–490
32. Landing BH, Kamoshita S (1970) Congenital hyperparathyroidism secondary to maternal hypoparathyroidism. J Pediatr 77:842–847
33. Forbes GB, Bryson MF, Manning J, et al (1972) Impaired calcium homeostasis in the infantile hypercalcemic syndrome. Acta Paediatr Scand 61:305–309
34. Norwood-Galloway A, Lebwohl M, Phelps RG, Raucher H (1987) Sucutaneous fat necrosis of the newborn with hypercalcemia. J Am Acad Dermatol 16:435–439
35. Drummond KN, Michael AF, Ulstrom RA, et al (1964) The blue diaper syndrome: familial hypercalcemia with nephrocalcinosis and indicanuria. Am J Med 37:928–948
36. Vido L, Carli M, Rizzoni G, Calo L, Dalla Palma P, Parenti A, Fusco F (1986) Congenital mesoblastic nephroma with hypercalcemia: pathogenetic role of prostaglandins. Am J Pediatr Hematol Oncol 8:149–152
37. Cooper L, Wertheimer J, Levey R, Brown E, Leboff M, Wilkinson R, Anast CS (1986) Severe primary hyperparathyroidism in a neonate with two hypercalcemic parents: management with parathyroidectomy and heterotopic autotransplantation. Pediatrics 78:263–268
38. Lutz P, Kane O, Pfersdorff A, Seiller F, Sauvage P, Levy JM (1986) Neonatal primary hyperparathyroidism: total parathyroidectomy with autotransplantation of cryopreserved parathyroid tissue. Acta Paediatr Scand 75:179–182
39. Page LA, Haddow JE (1987) Self-limited neonatal hyperparathyroidism in familial hypocalciuric hypercalcemia. J Pediatr 111:261–264
40. Kinder BK, Rasmussen H (1985) New applications of total parathyroidectomy and autotransplantation: use in proximal renal tubular dysfunction. World J Surg 9:156–164
41. Ross AJ III, Dale JK, Gunnells JC, Wells SA Jr (1979) Parathyroid transplantation: fate of a long-term allograft in man. Surgery 85:382–384

Current Status of Pancreatectomy for Persistent Idiopathic Neonatal Hypoglycemia Due to Islet Cell Dysplasia

R. M. Filler[1], M. J. Weinberg[4], E. Cutz[2], D. E. Wesson[1], and R. M. Ehrlich[3]

Summary

A series of 18 children suffering from persistent idiopathic neonatal hypoglycemia (PINH) is reported. Medical and surgical managements are described in detail. All patients subjected to surgery had failed medical treatment. These patients were divided into two groups: 1) 85% pancreatectomy leaving the uncinate process in situ, and 2) 95% pancreatectomy leaving a small rim of pancreatic tissue along the duodenum and the common bile duct. The spleen was preserved in all cases. Two out of 5 children of group 1 required further resection of the pancreas for persistent hypoglycemia and were converted to 95% pancreatectomy. Since 1981 95% pancreatectomy was exclusively employed. Only one patient required insulin for 3 weeks postoperatively. Histopathology and immunohistochemistry revealed islet cell dysplasia and islet cell nuclear hypertrophy in the majority of cases. 35% of the patients had focal adenomatosis. Better control of hypoglycemia is achieved by primary 95% pancreatectomy and, thus, 95% pancreatectomy is recommended as the initial procedure in the treatment of PINH.

Zusammenfassung

Es wird eine Serie von 18 Kindern mit persistierender, idiopathischer neonataler Hypoglykämie (PINH) vorgestellt. Konservative und chirurgische Behandlungen werden detailliert beschrieben. Bei allen Kindern, die operiert wurden, hatte die konservative Behandlung versagt. Diese Patienten wurden in 2 Gruppen eingeteilt: 1) 85%-Pankreatektomie unter Zurücklassung des Processus uncinatus und 2) 95%-Pankreatektomie unter Zurücklassung eines schmalen Saumes von Pankreasgewebe entlang Duodenum und Ductus choledochus. Die Milz wurde in allen Fällen erhalten; 2 Kinder aus Gruppe 1 mußten sich einer weiteren Pankreasresektion unterziehen und gelangten somit in Gruppe 2. Seit 1981 wird nur noch die 95%-Pankreatektomie durchgeführt. Nur 1 Patient benötigte Insulin für 3 Wochen nach der Operation. Histopathologie und Immunhistochemie ergaben eine Inselzelldysplasie und Inselzellkernhypertrophie in der Mehrzahl der Fälle. 35% hatten eine fokale Adenomatose. Eine bessere Kontrolle der Hypoglykämien wird durch die primäre 95%-Pankreatektomie erreicht, und deshalb wird die 95%-Pankreatektomie als primäre Operation zur Behandlung der PINH empfohlen.

Résumé

Les auteurs présentent une série de 18 enfants atteints d' hypoglycémie idiopathique néonatale persistante. Le traitement, tant médical que chirurgical est décrit en détails. Dans le cas de tous

[1]Department of Surgery,
[2]Department of Pathology, and
[3]Department of Endocrinology, Hospital for Sick Children Toronto, Ontario, Canada.
[4]University of Toronto, Toronto, Ontario, Canada.

Progress in Pediatric Surgery, Vol. 26
Gauderer and Angerpointner (Eds.)
© Springer-Verlag Berlin Heidelberg 1991

les patients ayant subi une intervention chirurgicale, le traitement médical avait échoué. Ces patients ont été répartis en deux groupes: 1) pancréatectomie à 85%, laissant en place le processus uncinatus pancreatis et 2) pancréatectomie à 95% laissant en place une étroite bordure de tissu pancréatique le long du duodénum et du canal cholédoque. La rate est restée en place dans tous les cas. Deux des enfants du groupe 1 ont dû subir une nouvelle résection du pancréas, l'hypoglycémie persistant, passant ainsi dans le groupe 2 des pancréatectomies à 95%. Depuis 1981, ce type d'intervention fut d'ailleurs le seul à être utilisé. Un seul patient eut besoin d'une administration d'insuline durant les trois semaines suivant l'intervention. Dans la majorité des cas, l'examen histopathologique et immunohistochimique révéla une dysplasie des îlots et une hypertrophie de leurs noyaux. 35% des patients présentaient une adénomatose focale. Le traitment de choix de l'hypoglycémie reste donc la pancréatectomie á 95% qui doit être le premier geste thérapeutique pour le traitement de l' hypoglycémie idiopathique néonatale persistante.

Introduction

Neonatal hypoglycemia occurs in approximately 4/1000 live term infants and in 16/1000 premature infants. Most cases respond well to intravenous infusion of glucose and resolve spontaneously [1]. There is, however, a rare subgroup who remain persistently hypoglycemic. Various terms have been used interchangeably to refer to these cases, including: "idiopathic" neonatal hypoglycemia, nesidioblastosis, islet cell dysplasia and idiopathic neonatal hyperinsulinism. We suggest that the correct terminology should be persistent idiopathic neonatal hypoglycemia (PINH) to describe the clinical presentation and islet cell dysplasia (ICD) to describe the pathology. Typically, patients have blood insulin levels' that, although they may be in the "normal range", are inappropriately elevated in the presence of a markedly decreased blood glucose [1]. Children with this abnormality are medical emergencies that require prompt investigation and aggressive treatment.

The etiology of this syndrome is unknown. Heitz et al. [2] suggested that the histological resemblance of nesidioblastic pancreata to those from immature fetuses had arisen as a result of inappropriate control during the earliest phases of endocrine pancreatic development. Whether this is due primarily to a genetic defect or is a result of external factors cannot be answered until more is known of the factors regulating fetal pancreatic development. There may be a genetic component with an autosomal recessive pattern suggested by the familial occurrence of PINH [3–6] and especially associated with familial endocrine adenomatosis [7].

In the past, PINH was frequently associated with severe long-term neurological disability. In recent years, early adequate control of blood glucose levels through both aggressive medical and surgical treatment has prevented these sequelae.

The diagnosis is generally easy to make. The babies are generally large and look like the infants of diabetic mothers. At the time of hypoglycemia the blood sugar is obviously low, the insulin levels inappropriately high, and free fatty acids and ketone bodies are both low. It should be emphasized that several laboratory determinations are usually necessary to establish the diagnosis [8].

Table 1. Patients requiring surgery for persistent idiopathic neonatal hypoglycemia

Patient	Sex	Age	Medical management			Surgery	Complications	Result
			i.v. Glucose	Diazoxide	Glucagon	Primary procedure		
1. DL	F	4 mos	×	×	×	85%	None	Died age 3 – pneumonia
2. AP	F	1 mo	×	×	×	85%	None	Well
3. SC	F	11 mos	×	×		85%	None	Well
4. GM	F	2 mos	×	×	×	85%	Recurrent hypoglycemia requiring 95%, then 100%	Requires insulin and pancreatic enzymes
5. MM	F	3 mos	×	×	×	85%	Recurrent hypoglycemia requiring 95%	Well
6. JM	F	5 mos	×	×	×	95%	CBD obstruction requiring choledochoduodenostomy	Well
7. MS	F	3 mos	×	×	×	95%	Wound infection	Well
8. CS	F	1 mo	×	×	×	95%	None	Well
9. WT	F	5 mos	×	×	×	95%	None	Well
10. TR	M	2 mos	×	×	×	95%	None	Well
11. AJ	F	5 wks	×	×	×	95%	Recurrent hypoglycemia requiring 98%	Well
12. PB	M	8 mos	×	×	×	95%	Hypoglycemic seizure, home on diazoxide	Not available for follow-up
13. TB	F	1 mo	×	×	×	95%	Intraoperative hypoglycemia requiring 98%; subsequent hyperglycemia requiring insulin for 9 weeks	Well
14. PS	F	1 mo	×	×	×	95%	None	Well
15. CE	M	1 mo	×	×	×	95%	None	Well
16. FD	F	4 mos	×	×	×	95%	None	Well
17. SL	F	1 mo	×	×	×	95%	None	Well
18. HS	F	1 mo	×	×	×	95%	None	Well

The Hospital for Sick Children, 12-Year-Experience

Between 1977 and 1989, 18 children with PINH were seen (Table 1). Some of the data from the first ten patients have been analyzed and reported previously [1, 9]. We include them in this report, since our current management is based on the results of the management of those patients, and follow-up data will be presented.

There were 15 females and 3 males. Eight were neonates, and the others presented between 2 months and 11 months of age. Twelve presented with seizures, one with irritability, one with blackout spells and four were asymptomatic. All patients were examined yearly, and growth parameters were measured, verbal and motor skills were assessed and blood sugar levels were evaluated.

Medical Management

The medical management at our institution involves a stepwise approach, based on the clinical picture and the blood sugar levels. Our first step involves the administration of intravenous dextrose. If the hypoglycemia cannot be controlled, then a central line is inserted and frequent feeds are started. Central venous lines allow much more reliable venous access and also continuous infusion of the hypertonic dextrose to maintain euglycemia while the doses of the next agents are adjusted. If the hypoglycemia persists, the next agent to be added is a glucagon infusion. The doses are stepped up as necessary. The last agent to be used is diazoxide. It has been our experience that the younger the child, the less effective is this agent. If the above measures fail to control the blood sugar, then surgery is undertaken.

Surgical Management

All patients subjected to surgery had failed medical management. The patients were divided retrospectively into two groups according to their initial operation. Group 1 was treated by 85% pancreatectomy, leaving the uncinate process in situ (Fig. 1a). Group 2 had a 95% pancreatectomy, leaving a small rim of pancreatic tissue along the duodenum and common bile duct (Fig. 1b). The spleen was preserved in all cases, either by ligation of the pancreatic branches of the splenic vessels or by mass ligation of the splenic artery (12 cases). In the latter situation the splenic blood flow was from the short gastric vessels. Radionuclide spleen scans were performed on all patients within 6 weeks of surgery and demonstrated normal splenic function in all.

Group I: 85% pancreatectomy. As noted in Table 1, cases 1–5 had 85% pancreatectomy. One patient suffered severe neurological impairment. This was due to poor preoperative blood sugar control and delay in instituting surgery. She was normoglycemic postoperatively and died of pneumonia at age 3. Two of the five children required a further resection and were converted to a 95% pancreatec-

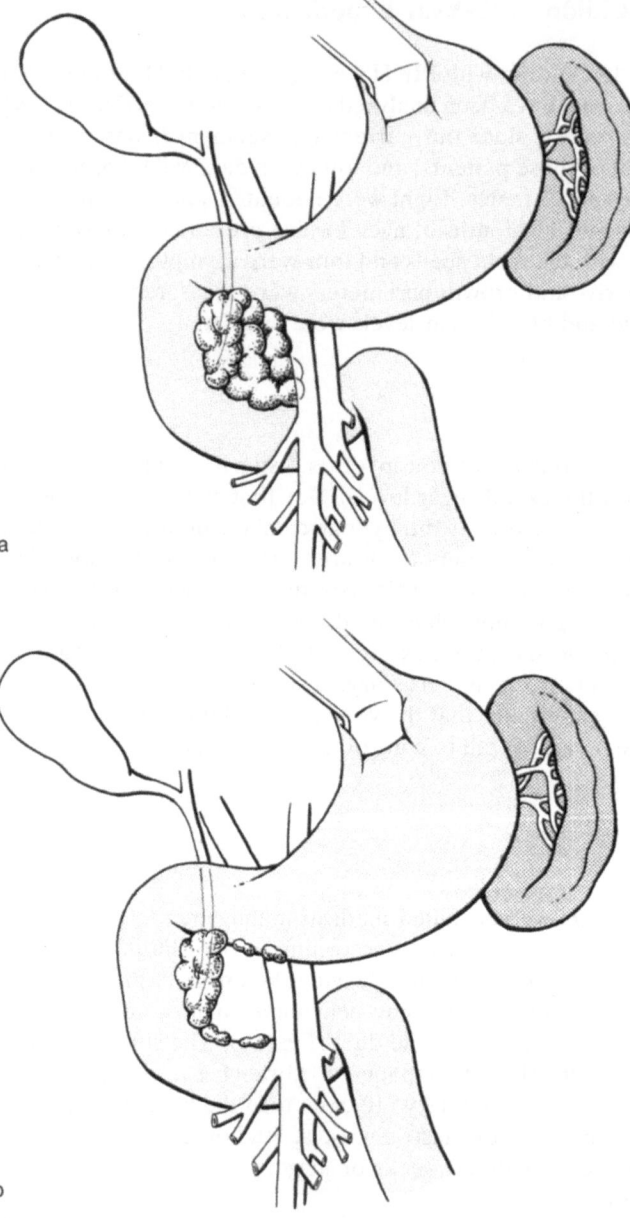

Fig. 1a, b. Result of 85% (**a**) and 95% (**b**) pancreatectomy

tomy. Both patients remained persistently hypoglycemic postoperatively. One underwent a second pancreatectomy 3 days later, and one underwent a second pancreatectomy 25 days postoperatively; the latter patient required subsequent total pancreatectomy 3 years later, due to intermittent seizures associated with recurrent hypoglycemic episodes. At laparotomy the pancreatic remnant was found to have regenerated to fill the C-loop of the duodenum. She now requires long-term pancreatic enzyme replacement and insulin. Except for the child who died of pneumonia the others are growing and developing normally.

Group II: 95% pancreatectomy. Because of the relatively high incidence of failure with lesser resections we have employed 95% pancreatectomy as the first surgical procedure since 1981. To date 13 children have had 95% pancreatectomy. The postoperative complications in this group included one mild would infection and one patient with persistent obstruction of the common bile duct, eventually requiring choledochoduodenostomy. Only one patient required insulin, which was discontinued 3 weeks postoperatively. All these patients were well at the most recent follow-up although case 12 had not been followed because the family resides outside of Canada. The 95% resection failed to control hypoglycemia in three children. One child had persistent hypoglycemia on the operating table and a near total pancreatectomy was performed (case 13). Similarly, a second child had recurrent hypoglycemia and a near total pancreatectomy was necessary (case 11) 10 months after the primary procedure. One child (case 12) required diazoxide postoperatively.

Pathology

Gross Findings

The pathological findings are summarized in Table 2 and Fig. 2. On gross examination, most resected pancreata showed no obvious abnormalities. However, in three patients a single whitish-tan nodule (< 1.0 cm) was identified either during surgery or later by the pathologist. In two cases the nodule was located on the surface of the pancreas, and in one case a 0.2-cm nodule embedded within the parenchyma was found after serial sectioning of the specimen. On microscopic examination, the nodule in each case was composed of islet cells mixed with exocrine elements, forming an area of focal adenomatosis (see Fig. 5a).

Histopathology and Immunohistochemistry

Islet Cell Dysplasia

On routine hematoxylin and eosin sections, abnormal distribution and disorganization of islets is not readily apparent, and immunostaining for islet cell hormones and/or other islet markers is necessary to demonstrate the lesion (Fig. 3a, b). These lesions comprise a set of changes including (a) loss of discrete centrilobular

Table 2. Summary of pathology findings in 18 patients

Patient	Pathology findings			
	ICD	NH	FA	DA
1. DL	+	+	+[a]	/
2. AP	+	++	+[a]	/
3. SC	+	+	/	/
4. GM	+	+	/	/
5. MM	+	++	+	/
6. JM	+	+++	/	/
7. MS	+	+++	+/	/
8. CS	+	+++	/	/
9. WT	+	/	/	+
10. TR	/	/	/	/
11. AJ	+	+++	/	/
12. PB	+	+	+	/
13. TB	+	++	/	+[b]
14. PS	+	++	/	/
15. CE	+	++	+	/
16. FD	+	+	/	/
17. SL	+	/	/	/
18. HS	+	+++	/	/

ICD, Islet cell dysplasia; NH, nuclear hypertrophy (polyploidy); FA, focal adenomatosis; DA, diffuse adenomatosis; +, present; /, not observed

[a] Visible nodule (0.2–0.7 cm)

[b] Pancreas hamartoma

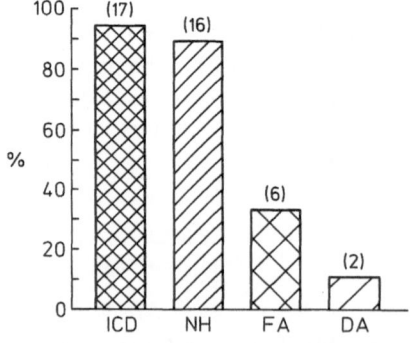

Fig. 2. Distribution of pathology findings in 18 patients with persistent idiopathic neonatal hypoglycemia. Numbers in parentheses represent numbers of patients. *ICD*, Islet cell dysplasia; *NH*, nuclear hypertrophy; *FA*, focal adenomatosis; *DA*, diffuse adenomatosis

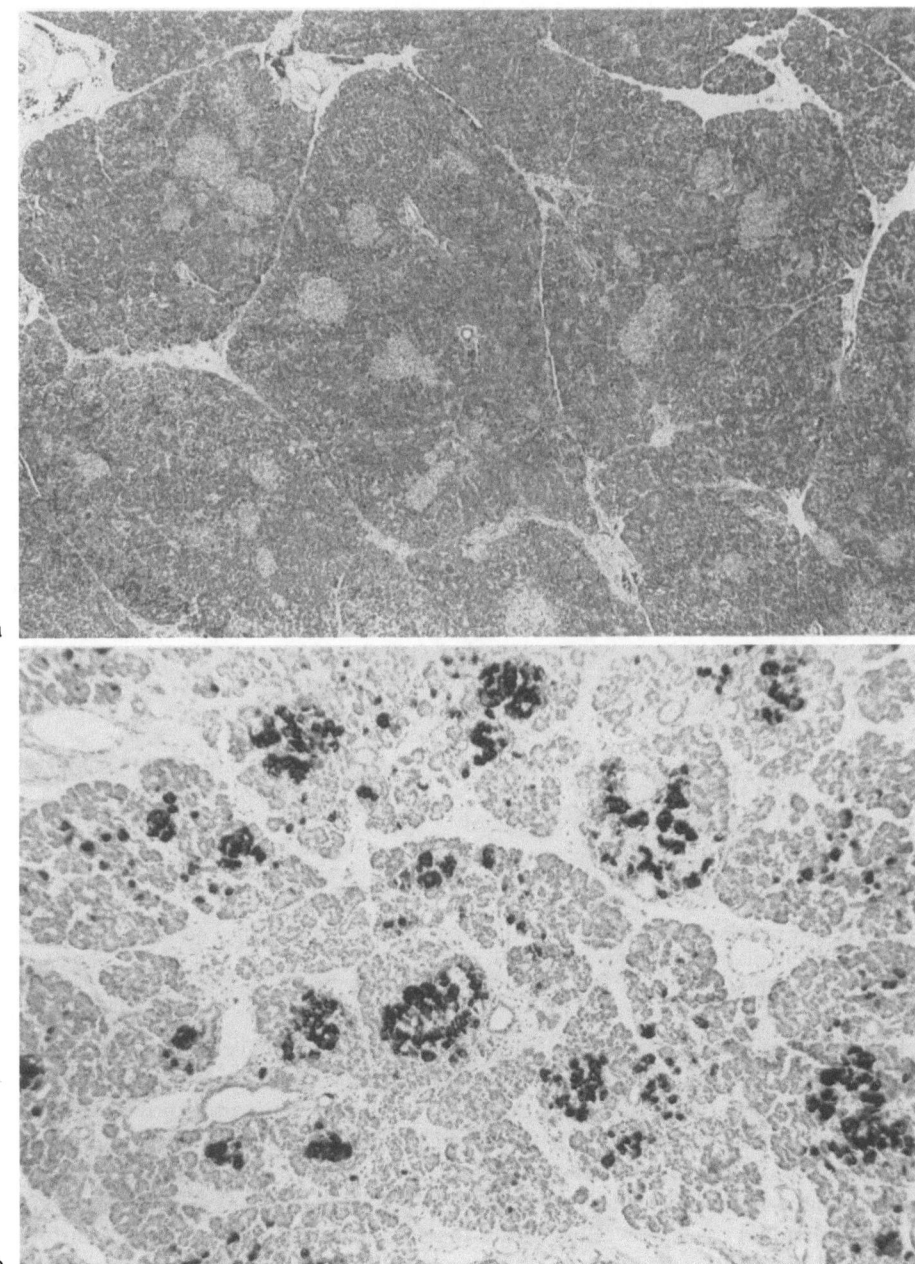

Fig. 3. a Low-magnification view of a section from patient 18, showing well-preserved exocrine tissue and several irregular islets of Langerhans *(pale areas)* in a routine H & E stain. × 25. **b** Similar field as in **a**, but immunostained with an antibody against insulin. Islet cells (darkly stained) show positive reaction, with "ragged" islet shape and distribution, i.e., poorly defined clusters. This abnormal distribution of islets is not apparent on a routine section. × 63

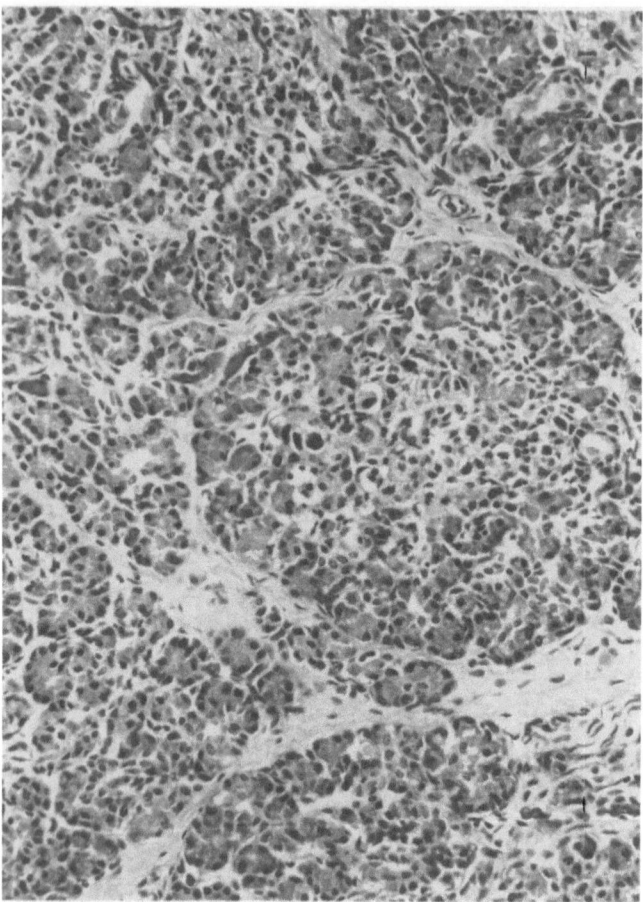

Fig. 4. Higher magnification of islet cells with large, irregular "dysplastic" nuclei, an additional feature of islet cell dysplasia (case 11). H & E, × 225

islet formation, (b) an increase in single and small endocrine cell clusters randomly distributed throughout exocrine tissue, (c) irregular islet cell contour ("ragged" islets) and (d) islet cell nuclear hypertrophy. Although it is not known whether these abnormalities are the basis for hypoglycemia, these lesions were found in the majority of cases and were not observed in the normal postnatal pancreas. Considerable variation in the extent and degree of these changes was noted between individual cases as well as within the same pancreas. In our series, diffuse abnormal distribution of islets was seen in the majority of cases (94%), with the exception of a single patient (case 10) in whom the endocrine pancreas appeared histologically normal.

Islet cell nuclear hypertrophy as evidenced by large polyploid nuclei (2–6 times greater than normal) is another distinctive feature of ICD (Fig. 4). In our

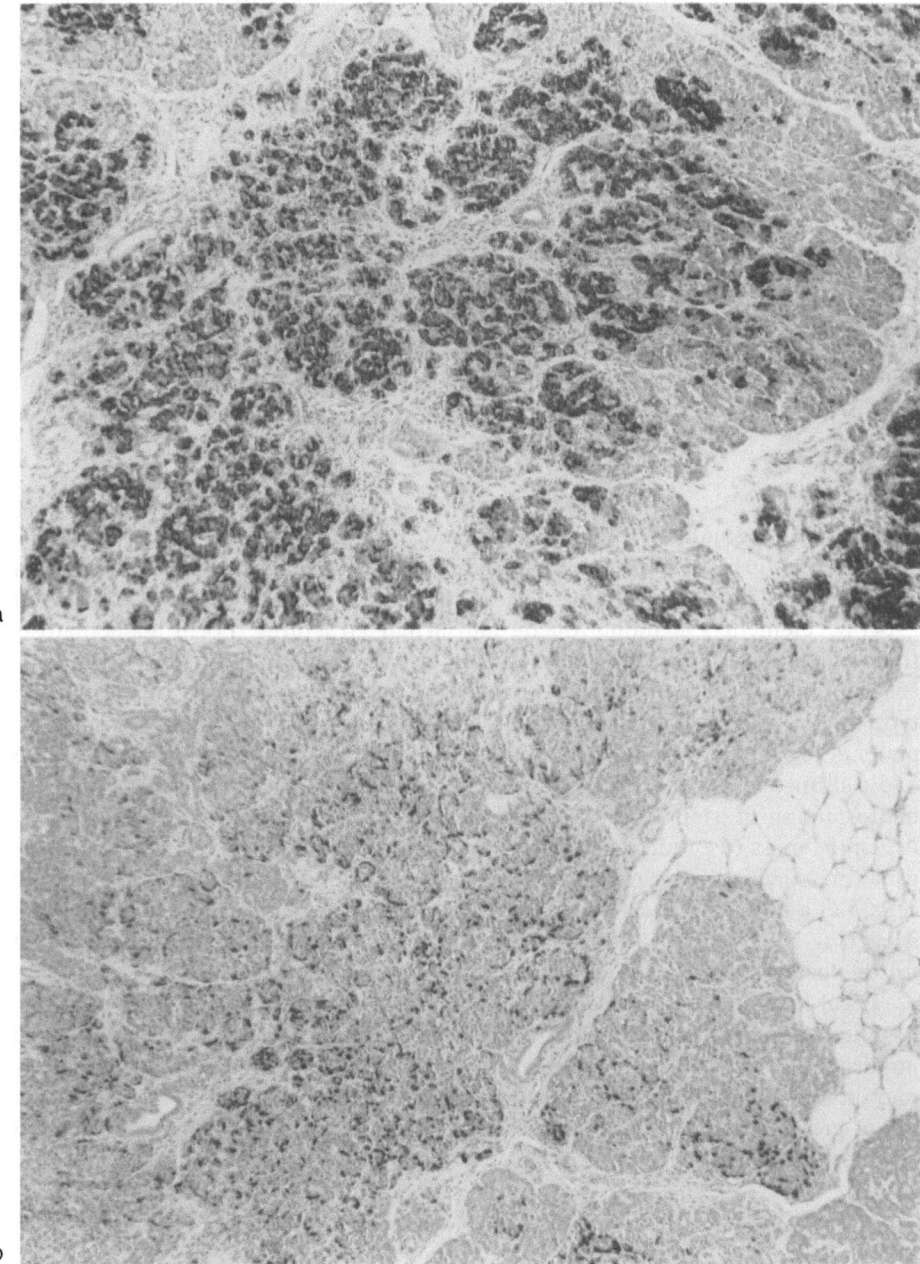

Fig. 5. a Area of focal adenomatosis (case 7) with closely packed aggregates of insulin-producing B cells. Immunostaining for insulin, × 63. **b** Section adjacent to that in **a**, immunostained for glucagon showing χ-cells at the periphery of B-cell aggregates, as in normal islets. × 63

series, islet cell nuclear hypertrophy was observed in 88% of cases, although the number and distribution of islet cells with large nuclei varied between cases (see Table 2 and Fig. 2). While in some cases only occasional cells with large nuclei were observed in a few islets, in others this change involved the majority of islets. The predominant islet cells with hypertrophic nuclei appear to be insulin-producing B cells (Fig. 4), but occasional somatostatin-immunopositive D cells have been shown to exhibit a similar change [10, 11]. On the other hand, glucagon-producing A cells do not appear to be affected. The presence of nuclear hypertrophy is generally considered a sign of cell hypertrophy and hyperfunction. In the case of islet cell dysplasia, this change most likely reflects hypersecretion of insulin and points to B cells as being the main abnormal element involved in this disorder. Furthermore, the finding of hypertrophic islet cell nuclei is a useful diagnostic marker of ICD, which is easily detected even on routinely stained sections (Fig. 4).

Adenomatosis

The term adenomatosis refers to localized or diffuse proliferation of islet cells which form a grossly and/or microscopically identifiable lesion (usually < 1 cm in diameter). Microscopically, this lesion consists of a mixture of endocrine and exocrine elements, including ductal and acinar structures. Focal adenomatosis (microadenomatosis) is distinguished from a true adenoma by its heterogeneous cell population, that of a true adenoma being made up exclusively of a single cell type (e.g., a true insulinoma is composed of B cells only). In our series, six of 17 patients (35%) were found to have focal adenomatosis and two patients (12%) had a diffuse lesion (see Table 2; Fig. 2). The notable features include areas of neoformation of islets from ductal elements and the presence of acinar cells between the mass of endocrine cells (Fig. 5). The islet cells, however, maintain their usual organization and arrangement, including peripheral placement of A and D cells; i.e. a nodule of focal adenomatosis is composed of a cluster of well-defined islets (Fig. 5). In cases with diffuse adenomatosis, the same changes as described for the localized form a affect a large portion of the pancreas.

Focal adenomatosis and diffuse adenomatosis are considered to be the most advanced lesions in the spectrum of islet cell dysplasia [10, 12, 13]. The practical implication is that cases with diffuse disorganization of islets without adenomatosis may potentially be amenable to nonsurgical treatment and may resolve as the infant grows older, whereas for focal or diffuse adenomatosis surgical resection remains the treatment of choice.

Discussion

Morphological changes in the endocrine pancreas of infants with PINH have been the subject of several recent studies and reviews [10–14]. Systematic immuno-histochemical studies, combined with electron microscopy, revealed several new findings, leading to revision of previous notions of the underlying islet cell abnormalities. A revised terminology, together with new pathologic criteria for morphological diagnosis of this disorder, has emerged. The previous term "nesidioblastosis" (neoformation of islets) has been replaced by "islet cell dysplasia", to highlight specific pathologic features and to differentiate them from normal developmental changes [10, 14]. The term islet cell dysplasia (endocrine cell dysplasia, nesidiodysplasia) encompasses a wide range of lesions which can be encountered singly or in combination, including diffuse abnormal distribution and disorganization of islets, islet cell and islet hypertrophy and diffuse or focal proliferation of islet cells (adenomatosis) [10, 12, 13]. Thus, while there is no general agreement on terminology, it is widely acknowledged that this rather uniform clinical entity is associated with heterogeneous pathologic changes. It is also becoming more evident that abnormal regulation of insulin secretion rather than true neoplasia is the underlying abnormality.

The degree and duration of hypoglycemia tolerated by the CNS without permanent neurologic sequelae appear to very widely. Some infants can withstand numerous episodes without significant deficit, while others with borderline hypoglycemia sustain severe deficits early in their course [15]. One factor that probably influences the susceptibility of the CNS to hypoglycemia is the availability of alternative substrates such as ketone bodies, which the brain can use when glucose is scarce. When hypoglycemia is associated with a relative hyperinsulinemia the levels of insulin inhibit lipolysis and prevent the formation of ketone bodies. As a result, infants with this cause of hypoglycemia are more apt to develop permanent neurologic deficits than those with ketotic hypoglycemia.

Since 1934, when Graham and Hartman [17] resected 80%–90% of the pancreas in a 1-year-old child with hypoglycemia, surgery has gained an increasingly important place in the therapy of hypoglycemia secondary to various pancreatic disorders [18]. As recently as 17 years ago, persistent neonatal hypoglycemia was associated with neurologic and developmental morbidity in more than 50% of cases [15], regardless of the extent of pancreatic resection. Thomas et al. [16] reviewed 66 patients with intractable hypoglycemia and found that the delay between diagnosis and surgery had been shorter in those with normal mental development than in those with retarded postoperative and mental development. The mean delay in patients with normal postoperative development was 6 months compared with 10 months in patients with retardation, but the difference was not statistically significant. The rather long delays before surgery may explain why the overall incidence of mental retardation in the Thomas series was 52%.

When a pancreatectomy is undertaken, splenectomy is not advised. The increased incidence of sepsis following splenectomy in infants and children is well known, and the same procedure when accompanied by PINH seems to carry an even greater risk. A review of 19 cases where spenectomy was undertaken disclosed seven patients (37%) who suffered infectious complications, with four cases of overwhelming postsplenectomy sepsis reported [19]. An 85%–95% pancreatic resection can be carefully performed with all pancreatic tributaries of the splenic artery and vein ligated, thus preserving normal splenic perfusion.

Alternatively, the main splenic vessels may be ligated with careful preservation of the short gastric vessels, which will maintain splenic viability.

Early reports of idiopathic neonatal hypoglycemia suggested that a subtotal resection of approximately 75% (to the level of the superior mesenteric artery) should be performed [20, 21]. More recent evidence indicates that more extensive resection is necessary to eliminate hypoglycemia and decrease the high failure rate with neurologic sequelae following the traditional operation [1, 15, 18].

Clearly, if a discrete adenoma is found, then it must be removed. However, in almost all cases no gross lesion is seen, and a decision must be made as to how extensive a resection should be done [1]. The extent of pancreatectomy required to achieve the euglycemic state has been debated. Preoperatively, the clinical presentation, serum glucose and insulin levels, and the response to diazoxide are of no predictive value as to the cause of hyperinsulinism [8]. Microscopic examination of frozen biopsy material obtained during the operative procedure when the pancreas is grossly normal is generally inadequate to define the underlying pathologic process [8]. Thus, the decision about the extent of resection is a difficult one, and the surgeon must be guided solely by his or her philosophy and experience [8].

Martin et al. [19] reviewed the complete literature in 1984, which consisted of 181 cases. In the group that underwent less than 80% pancreatectomy, almost half of the patients required additional medical therapy to control persistent or recurrent hypoglycemia. In addition, one quarter required further pancreatectomy because of persistent symptoms refractory to medical therapy [22–51]. These data encouraged most surgeons to pursue a more aggressive initial surgical approach to this condition. When 85%–95% pancreatectomy has been performed, control of hypoglycemia has improved markedly. Of 63 cases reported in the literature, reoperation was required in only 8%, and only 20% required additional medical treatment [3, 19, 23, 29, 37, 45, 52–60]. Diabetes was not a significant complication.

We have previously reviewed our own experience, and in a small consecutive series we have compared pancreatectomy in the treatment of this disease [1, 9]. These results are reviewed earlier in this paper. Since there was no difference in operative morbidity, mortality or long-term results (given that two of the five patients initially undergoing 85% pancreatectomy subsequently had more extensive resections) and because there is better control of hypoglycemia with more extensive resection, we now recommend 95% pancreatectomy as the initial procedure of choice for these patients.

References

1. Langer KC, Filler RM, Wesson DE, Sherwood G, Cutz E (1984) Surgical management of persistent neonatal hypoglycemia due to islet cell dysplasia. J Pediatr Surg 19(6):786–790
2. Heitz PU, Kloppel G, Hacki WH, Polak JM, Pearse AG (1977) Nesidioblastosis: the pathologic basis of persistent hyperinsulinemic hypoglycemia in infants. Diabetes 26:632–642

3. Misugi K, Misugi N, Sotos J, Smith B (1970) The pancreatic islet of infants with severe hypoglycemia. Arch Pathol 89:208–220
4. Woo D, Scopes JW, Polak JM (1976) Idiopathic hypoglycemia in sibs with morphological evidence of nesidioblastosis of the pancreas. Arch Dis Child 51:528–531
5. Sovik O, Fevang FO, Finne PH (1978) Familial nesidioblastosis (abstract) In: proceedings of the European Society for Paediatric Research, Turku, Finland
6. Landau H, Perlman M, Meyer S, Isachsohn M, Krausz M, Mayan H, Lijovetzky G, Schiller M (1982) Persistent neonatal hypoglycemia due to hyperinsulinism: medical aspects. Pediatrics 70:440–446
7. Vance JE, Stoll RW, Kitabchi AE, Williams RH, Wood FC Jr (1969) Nesidioblastosis in familial endocrine adenomatosis. JAMA 207:1679–1682
8. Moosa AR, Baker L, Lavell-Jones M (1987) Hypoglycemic syndrome in infancy and childhood: a surgeon's perspective. West J Med 146:585–588
9. Jacobs DG, Haka-Ikse K, Wesson DE, Filler RM, Sherwood G (1986) Growth and development in patients operated on for islet cell dysplasia. J Pediatr Surg 21 (12):1184–1189
10. Jaffe R, Hashida Y, Yunis EJ (1980) Pancreatic pathology in hyperinsulinemic hypoglycemia of infancy. Lab Invest 42:356–365
11. Drut R, Drut RM (1987) An immunohistochemical study of islet cells with macronuclei in infancy. Pediatr Pathol 7:585–591
12. Kloppel G, Heitx PHU (1984) Nesidioblastosis: a clinical entity with heterogeneous lesions of the pancreas. In: Falkner S, Hakanson R, Sundler F (eds) Evolution and tumor pathology of the neuroendocrine system. Elsevier Science, Amsterdam, pp 349–370
13. Kloppel G, Sajons I, Schulte H, Nizze H, Andermatt HJ, Heitz PHU (1986) Focal and diffuse nesidioblastosis and persistent hyperinsulinemic hypoglycemia: a morphologic analysis of 12 patients. Pathologe 7:266–275
14. Gould VE, Memoli VA, Dardi LE, Gould NS (1983) Nesidiodysplasia and nesidioblastosis of infancy: structural and functional correlations with the syndrome of hyperinsulinemic hypoglycemia. Pediatr Pathol 1:7–31
15. Harken AH, Filler AM, Avruskin TW, Crigler SF (1971) The role of total pancreatectomy in the treatment of unremitting hypoglycemia of infancy. J Pediatr Surg 6:284–289
16. Thoms CG jr, Underwood LE, Carney CN, Dolcourt JL, Whitt JJ (1977) Neonatal and infantile hypoglycemia due to insulin excess: new aspects of diagnosis and surgical management. Ann Surg 185:505–517
17. Graham EA, Hartmann AF (1934) Subtotal resection of pancreas for hypoglycemia. Surg Gynecol Obstet 59:474–479
18. Kramer JL, Bell MJ, DeSchryer K, Bower RJ, Ternberg JL, White NH (1982) Clinical and histologic indications for extensive pancreatic resection in nesidioblastosis. Am J Surg 143:116–119
19. Martin LW, Ryckman FC, Sheldon CA (1984) Experience with 95% pancreatectomy and splenic salvage for neonatal nesidioblastosis. Ann Surg 200:355–362
20. Hamilton JP, Baker L, Kaye R, et al (1967) Subtotal pancreatectomy in the management of severe persistent idiopathic hypoglycemia in children. Pediatrics 39:49–54
21. Fonkalsrud EW, Trout HH, Lippe B, La Franchi S, Oakake C (1974) Idiopathic hypoglycemia in infancy: surgical management. Arch Surg 108:801–804
22. Aynsley-Green A, Polack JM, Bloom SR, et al (1981) Nesidioblastosis of the pancreas: definition of the syndrome and the management of the severe neonatal hyperinsulinemic hypoglycemia. Arch Dis Child 56:496–508
23. Schwarts SS, Rich BH, Lucky AW, et al (1979) Familial nesidioblastosis: severe neonatal hypoglycemia in two families. J Pediatr 95:44–53
24. Kushner RS, Lemli L, Smith DW (1963) Zinc glucagon in the management of idiopathic hypoglycemia. J Pediatr 1111–1115
25. Aynsley-Green A (1982) The regulation of blood glucose concentration. Clin Endocrinol Metab 11:159–194
26. Ernesti M, Mitchell ML, Ragen MS, Gilboa (1965) Control of hypoglycemia with diazoxide and human growth hormone. Lancet 1:628–630

27. Griffith JE, Jackson RL, Janes RG (1951) Action of alloxan on a hypoglycemic infant. Pediatrics 7:616–622
28. Greenlee RF, White RR (1952) Phillip chronic hypoglycemia in an infant treated by subtotal pancreatectomy. JAMA 149 (3):272–273
29. Gross RE (1953) Hypoglycemia. In: Gross RE (ed) The surgery of infancy and childhood. Saunders, Philadelphia, pp 574–587
30. McQuarrie R (1954) Idiopathic spontaneous occurring hypoglycemia in infants. Am J Dis Child 4:399–428
31. Conn JW, Seltzer HS (1955) Spontaneous hypoglycemia. Am J Med 19:460–478
32. Porter MR, Frantz VK (1956) Tumors associated with hypoglycemia-pancreatic and extra-pancreatic. Am J Med 21:944–961
33. Cochrane WA, Payne WW, Simkiss MJ, Woolf LI (1956) Familial hypoglycemia precipitated by amino acids. J Clin Invest 35:411–423
34. Farber S (1959) Clinical pathological conference. The Children's Medical Center, Boston. Pediatrics 54:116
35. Hawath MB, Coodin FJ (1960) Idiopathic spontaneous hypoglycemia in children. Pediatrics 25:748–765
36. Traisman HS, Steiner MM, Ziering W (1962) Spontaneous hypoglycemia treated by partial pancreatectomy. Ann Surg 156:743–748
37. Cunningham GC (1964) Tolbutamide tolerance in hypoglycemic children. Am J Dis Child 107:417–423
38. Drash AL (1966) The use of diazoxide in the treatment of hypoglycemia (abstract). J Pediatr 69:970
39. Peters HS (1965) Pancreatic resection for hypoglycemia in childhood. Am J Surg 110:198
40. Frasier SD, Smith FG, Nash A (1965) The use of glucagon-gel in idiopathic spontaneous hypoglycemia of infancy. Pediatrics 35:120–123
41. Griese GG, Wenzel FJ (1965) Leucine-sensitive hypoglycemia treated with long-acting epinephrine. Pediatrics 35:709–712
42. McFarland JO, Gillett FS, Zwemer RF (1965) Total pancreatectomy for hyperinsulinism in infants. Surgery 57:313–318
43. Peters HE, Stanten A (1965) Pancreatic resection for hypoglycemia in children. Am J Surg 110:198–202
44. Harken AH, Filler RM, Avrusking TW, Crigler JF (1971) The role of "total" pancreatectomy in the treatment of unremitting hypoglycemia of infancy. J Pediatr Surg 6:284–289
45. Fonkalsrud EW, Trout HH, Lippe B, et al (1974) Idiopathic hypoglycemia in infancy. Arch Surg 108:801–804
46. Dahms BB, Lippe BM, Dakake C, et al (1976) The occurrence in a neonate of a pancreatic adenoma with nesidioblastosis in the tumor. Am J Clin Pathol 65:462–466
47. Woo D, Scopes JW, Polak JM (1976) Idiopathic hypoglycemia in sibs with morphological evidence of nesidioblastosis on the pancreas. Arch Dis Child 51:528–531
48. Habbick BF, Cram RW, Miller KR (1977) Neonatal hypoglycemia resulting from islet cell adenomatosis. Am J Dis Child 131:210–212
49. Falkmer S, Sovik O, Vidnes J (1981) Immunohistochemical morphometric and clinical studies of the pancreatic islets in infants with persistent neonatal hypoglycemia of familial type with hyperinsulinism and nesidioblastosis. Acta Biol Med Germ 40:39–54
50. Kramer JL, Bell MJ, DeSchryver K, et al (1982) Clinical and histologic indications for extensive pancreatic resection in nesidioblastosis. Am J Surg 143:116–119
51. Moazam F, Rodgers BM, Talbert JL, Rosenbloom AL (1982) Near total pancreatectomy in persistent infantile hypoglycemia. Arch Surg 117:1151–1154
52. Wangensteen OH (1937) Surgical diseases of the pancreas with special reference to cysts, acute pancreatic necrosis, and hyperinsulinism. Minn Med 19:566–567
53. White RR (1953) Organic hyperinsulinism. South Med J 16:150–174
54. Crowder WL, MacLaren NK, Gutberlet RL, et al (1976) Neonatal pancreas B-cell hyperplasia: report of a case with failure of diazoxide and benefit of early subtotal pancreatectomy. Pediatrics 57:897–900

55. Ravitch MM, Welch KJ, Benson CD, et al (eds) (1979) The pancreas. In: Pediatric surgery. Yearbook Medical, Chicago, pp 857–868
56. Knight J, Garvin PJ, Danis RK, et al. (1980) Nesidioblastosis in children. Arch Surg 115:880–882
57. Schiller M, Krausz M, Meyer S, et al (1980) Neonatal hyperinsulinism surgical and pathologic considerations. J Pediatr Surg 15:16–20
58. Lloyd RV, Caceres V, Warner FCS, Gilbert EF (1981) Islet cell adenomatosis. Arch Pathol Lab Med 105:198–202
59. Gairdner D, Robinson R (1978) Persistent neonatal hypoglycemia due to glucagon deficiency. Arch Dis Child 53:422–424
60. Baker L, Kaye R, Root AW, Prasad ALN (1968) Diazoxide treatment of idiopathic hypoglycemia of infancy. J Pediatr 71:494–505

Surgery for Nesidioblastosis –
Indications, Treatment and Results

B. Willberg[1] and E. Müller†

Summary

Nesidioblastosis is a life-threatening form of hypoglycemia that starts during the neonatal period in most cases and is caused by hyperinsulinism. Its diagnostic criteria are an extremely high demand for carbohydrates (more than 15 g/kg/day), an inadequately high plasma insulin level, and an inhibited production of ketone bodies. This acute, life-threatening hypoglycemia requires immediate intensive-care treatment. The most important aim of continuous therapy is the prevention of irreversible brain damage. This cannot be reliably avoided by conservative treatment (increased carbohydrate supply, diazoxide administration). Therefore, surgical treatment consisting in subtotal pancreatectomy is becoming increasingly important. The reduction of hormone-producing tissue resolves hyperinsulinism and apparently enables the onset of physiological regulatory mechanisms. Surgical strategy and results in 12 children who underwent surgery for nesidioblastosis are described.

Zusammenfassung

Die Nesidioblastose ist eine lebensbedrohliche, meist in der Neugeborenenperiode einsetzende, hyperinsulinismusbedingte Hypoglykämieform. Ihre diagnostischen Kriterien sind ein extrem hoher Kohlenhydratbedarf (über 15 g/kg/Tag), ein inadäquat hoher Plasmainsulinspiegel und eine gehemmte Ketonkörperbildung. Die akute, lebensbedrohliche Unterzuckerung bedarf sofortiger intensiv-therapeutischer Maßnahmen. Zentrales Ziel jeder Dauertherapie ist die Verhinderung irreparabler Hirnschäden. Diese lassen sich durch konservative Therapie (erhöhte Kohlenhydratzufuhr, Diazoxid) nicht zuverlässig vermeiden. Daher gewinnt die chirurgische Behandlung in Form der subtotalen Pankreassekretion zunehmend an Bedeutung. Diese führt über eine Reduktion des hormonproduzierenden Gewebes zur Beseitigung des Hyperinsulinismus und ermöglicht so offenbar das Ingangkommen physiologischer Regelmechanismen. Dargestellt werden die Operationstaktik und -technik sowie die Ergebnisse bei 12 Kindern, die wegen Nesidioblastose pankreasreseziert wurden.

Résumé

La nésidioblastose est une forme très dangereuse d'hypoglycémie, survenant le plus souvent durant la période néonatale et causée par une hyperinsulinie. Le critère diagnostique est un besoin extrêmement élevé en hydrates de carbone (plus de 15 g/kg/jour), un taux d'insuline trop élevé dans le plasma et une inhibition de la production de cétones. L'hypoglycémie aigue, extrêmement dangereuse, exige une traitement immédiat et intensif. Le but majeur de la thérapeutique continue est de prévenir un dommage cérébral irréversible. Le traitement conservateur (augmen-

---

[1] Department of Pediatric Surgery, Center for Operative Medicine, University of Düsseldorf, Moorenstraße 5, D-4000 Düsseldorf 1 (W), FRG.

tation de l'apport en hydrates de carbone, administration de diazoxide) n'est pas une garantie suffisante. Le traitement chirurgical, donc la pancréatectomie subtotale, prend de plus en plus d'importance. La réduction des tissus producteurs d'hormones résoud le problème de l'hyper-insulinie et met en place des mécanismes régulateurs physiologiques. La stratégie chirurgicale et les résultats obtenus dans le cas de 12 enfants ayant subi une intervention chirurgicale pour né-sidioblastose sont alors rapportés.

Introduction

Nesidioblastosis is a severe, continuous form of hypoglycemia usually occurring in the neonatal period that is caused by hyperinsulinism and leads to death when un-treated. The disease appears spontaneously in most cases, but autosomal reces-sive inheritance is considered possible in some cases with familial occurrence. The pathogenesis has not yet been fully clarified. The underlying pathological anatom-ical findings are inconsistent and their interpretation is somewhat controversial. It is not even clear whether the disease has one cause or whether various distur-bances result in a relatively homogeneous clinical picture.

The term "nesidioblastosis" was introduced by Laidlaw in 1938 for a diffuse in-crease of pancreatic islet cells as found in newborns with severe hypoglycemia. Today there is doubt whether a persistent formation of fetal B cells from the duc-tule epithelia of the exocrine pancreas independent from the Langerhans islets is the underlying pathophysiological mechanism [5]. Recent immunohistological investigations have shown that all endocrine elements of the pancreas exhibit qualitative and quantitative deviations from normal, although to different extents and in different combinations. However, an anomalous numerical relation between insulin- and somatostatin-producing cells is widely accepted; this is normally 2:1, but it is 5:1 in nesidioblastosis. Likewise, the B cells show signs of increased ac-tivity, in contrast to the D cells, which are clearly smaller and possess fewer granules. Further investigations are needed to determine the extent to which the uncontrolled release of insulin in nesidioblastosis results from a lack of counter-acting mechanisms. Our present knowledge is used therapeutically, however, in as much as the administration of somatostatin favorably affects threatening hypo-glycemia, which cannot be controlled by glucose administration alone [1, 8].

Clinical Picture

The clinical symptoms of nesidioblastosis begin mostly in the neonatal period, often as early as in the first hour of life, with centrally induced respiratory distur-bances, convulsions and cyanosis. The situation is usually so threatening that transferral to a pediatric intensive-care unit is mandatory. Serum glucose can drop to unmeasurably low levels. Death follows quickly if the condition remains un-treated.

When the life-threatening situation is under control, the aim of further treat-ment must be the permanent control of recurring hypoglycemia; otherwise, severe irreversible brain damage with general retardation and cerebral convulsions is the consequence. This is probably due to a decrease or lack of ketone bodies, which are essential for brain development.

Carcassone et al. [3] differentiated between the more common infant type of nesidioblastosis and a childhood type which does not become manifest until several months of age. Laboratory data and prognosis are similar to those for the infant type. The reasons for the late manifestation remain unknown. It may represent a milder form temporarily compensated by alimentary influences. It must be kept in mind that hypoglycemia as low as 30 mg% serum glucose may remain asymptomatic in infants [3].

In some cases spontaneous interruption of hypoglycemic states between the first and fourth year of life is observed. There are no prognostic criteria that allow an estimation of when and whether the endocrine pancreatic function normalizes.

Diagnosis

The following criteria are important for the diagnosis of insulin-induced hypoglycemia in infants and children:

- The hypoglycemia is always severe and lasts several hours.
- More than 15 g/kg/day of carbohydrates are necessary for normalization of serum glucose.
- The serum insulin level is too high with respect to serum glucose (glucose/insulin ratio less than 2).
- Serum ketone body levels are low.

These parameters should be measured as soon as possible; provocation tests for diagnosis must be avoided because of the extreme risk to the newborn. Based on the experience gathered by the nesidioblastosis group of our pediatric clinic, the amount of carbohydrates required for normalization of serum glucose is of particular diagnostic importance [2].

Treatment

Due to the high standard of pediatric intensive care, the treatment of life-threatening hypoglycemia is generally successful. It comprises high-dose parenteral glucose administration with serum glucose monitoring every 15 min and, if necessary, administration of somatostatin at an average dose of a 250 µg/1.73 m^2 body surface per hour [12].

Long-term therapy of nesidioblastosis is far more problematic; its central aim is to avoid irreversible brain damage. Medical treatment of recurrent hypoglycemia alone, usually with diazoxide, is normally insufficient.

For this reason, surgical treatment in the form of subtotal pancreatectomy is being increasingly favored. This resolves the hyperinsulinism by reducing the amount of hormone-producing tissue, making it possible for the physiological regulatory mechanisms to function. However, the 80% pancreatectomy used until the early 1970s turned out to be ineffective, since it provided only temporary improvement, soon followed by recurrences. Today, the 95% pancreatectomy has been established as the method of choice, leading to satisfactory results. Recurrences are rare. Hyperglycemic states still existing postoperatively are often temporary and may be compensated by diet in most cases. In contrast to the preoperative course, more pronounced postoperative hypoglycemia is easily controlled with diazoxide. It can therefore be assumed that surgical reduction of endocrine pancreatic tissue is prerequisite to effective medical therapy [6, 10, 11].

Surgery

Surgery is indicated as soon as possible after the diagnosis of nesidioblastosis has been established. Islet-cell adenoma, which must be considered in the differential diagnosis only in older children, also requires surgical treatment.

The surgical strategy of subtotal pancreatectomy for nesidioblastosis should take the following points into account. Clear access is best achieved by bilateral transverse upper abdominal laparotomy. For exclusion of ectopic pancreatic tissue the entire small intestine should be inspected; a Meckel's diverticulum deserves particular attention. Following opening of the bursa omentalis, the pancreas is explored carefully for islet-cell tumors; Kocher's maneuver greatly facilitates the exposure of the region of the pancreatic head. The spleen should be preserved whenever possible, since otherwise an inexcusably high rate of septic complications must be expected.

Technically, pancreatectomy begins with mobilization of the pancreatic tail, which might be difficult because this region is quite delicate in infancy. Careful dissection and ligation of small arteries and veins between the pancreatic and splenic vessels follows; great care must be taken to maintain the pancreas intact in order to avoid intraoperative efflux of pancreatic juice. The area of venous confluence is particularly problematic, since the pancreas is often adhered to it. The pancreas should not be resected at this level since, as mentioned above, an 80% resection is not a definitely curative measure and reoperation is often required. The pancreas should instead be excised near the duodenum, attention being paid to the common bile duct. The uncinate processus, which is usually enlarged, is also excised.

Postoperative care comprises parenteral nutrition for 1 week, a 10-day course of antibiotic therapy to prevent catheter sepsis, and frequent measurement of serum glucose levels to estimate the insulin requirement. The current tendency is to control postoperative hyperglycemia by reduced glucose administration at about 8–10 g/kg/day [7, 9].

Our Series

From 1976 to 1985, 12 infants and children underwent subtotal pancreatectomy for nesidioblastosis at the Department of Pediatric Surgery of the University of Düsseldorf. Ten patients were followed up for 9 months to 10 years postoperatively.

Siblings suffering from hypoglycemia were observed in three instances. Two of them have died; the third sibling still has episodes of hypoglycemia at the age of 15 years and is mentally retarded.

Nine children presented with symptoms (cyanosis, apneic spells, hypotonia, tremors, tonic-clonic convulsions) immediately after delivery; three children fell ill at the ages of 4, 6, and 7 months respectively.

Relative hyperinsulinism was shown in all cases. The compensatory carbohydrate requirement was between 18 and 31 g/kg/day. Only one of the ten children who received diazoxide prior to surgery was asymptomatic at operation on the 13th day. All other children presented with symptomatic hypoglycemia despite administration of high-dose carbohydrates and diazoxide.

Preoperatively, serum glucose was stabilized by administration of somatostatin for a maximum of 5 days in five instances. Two infants, operated on at the 16th and 26th day of life respectively, were treated exclusively with somatostatin.

Five children presented preoperatively with marked, two with severe, psychomotor retardation. Four of these children required anticonvulsant therapy. Only one of the children, whose development corresponded to its age, required anticonvulsants (Table 1).

Four infants underwent subtotal pancreatectomy during the first 4 weeks of life. Only three children were operated on beyond the first year of life, at 16, 31, and 40 months respectively. Technically, surgical reduction of hormone-producing pancreatic tissue was carried out as a four-fifths resection in two cases and as a seven-eighths resection in the remaining cases. Pathohistological, immunocytochemical, and electron-microscopical examinations confirmed the preoperative diagnosis in all cases.

Intraoperative complications included accidental lesion of the splenic vein in three instances; it was reconstructed in one case and ligated in the other two. The spleen was preserved in every case. The remaining part of the pancreas was closed using prolene-U sutures and additional Z sutures without additional ligation of the pancreatic duct. No leakage was observed.

Postoperative surgical problems occurred only once, in the form of mechanical ileus which necessitated relaparotomy 5 months following pancreatectomy. During the same session a hiatal hernia was repaired by means of a fundoplication. The pancreatic remnant was unsuspicious. Because of postoperative sepsis in four children, probably due to the central venous catheters, routine antibiotic therapy was conducted for 10 days.

Ten children required insulin for 1–76 days postoperatively for transitory hyperglycemia. None of the children, however, developed insulin-dependent diabetes mellitus. Five of the children have a borderline or pathological glucose tolerance. Insufficiency of the exocrine pancreas was not observed in any case.

Table 1. Time of onset, conservative preoperative treatment, preoperative state, and age at operation of 12 children with nesidioblastosis

Patient/sex	Time of onset	Conservative treatment	Preoperative state	Age at operation
MM/F	Delivery	Diazoxide	Age correspondent	13 days
SB /F	Delivery	Diazoxide	Age correspondent	16 days
BS /M	Delivery	Somatostatin	Age correspondent	16 days
KS /F	Delivery	Somatostatin	Age correspondent	26 days
WC/F	Delivery	Diazoxide, anticonvulsants	Severe retardation	13 weeks
LS /F	Delivery	Diazoxide	Age correspondent	15 weeks
TA /F	Delivery	Diazoxide, anticonvulsants	Retardation	8 months
SD /M	6 months	Diazoxide, somatostatin	Age correspondent	10 months
BM /M	Delivery	Diazoxide, anticonvulsants	Age correspondent	12 months
SD /F	Delivery	Diazoxide	Retardation	16 months
FM /M	4 months	Diazoxide, anticonvulsants	Severe retardation	31 months
NC /M	7 months	Diazoxide, somatostatin, anticonvulsants	Retardation	40 months

Table 2. Preoperative state, age at operation and results of subtotal pancreatectomy in 12 children with nesidioblastosis

Patient/sex	Preoperative state	Age at operation	Postoperative results	Age at follow-up
MM/F	Age correspondent	13 days	Age correspondent, normal glucose tolerance	5 years
SB /F	Age correspondent	16 days	Age correspondent, sent to school, borderline glucose tolerance	7 years
BS /M	Age correspondent	16 days	Age correspondent, borderline glucose tolerance	18 months
KS /F	Age correspondent	26 days	Age correspondent	9 months
WC/F	Severe retardation	13 weeks	Normoglycemia, convulsions	Discharge from hospital
LS /F	Age correspondent	15 weeks	Age correspondent, pathological glucose tolerance	3.5 years
TA /F	Retardation	8 months	Age correspondent, pathological glucose tolerance	2 years, 7 mos
SD /M	Age correspondent	10 months	Age correspondent	5 years
BM /M	Age correspondent	12 months	Age correspondent, sent to school	10 years
SD /F	Retardation	16 months	Retardation, normoglycemia	2 years, 5 mos
FM /M	Severe retardation	31 months	Severe retardation, no normoglycemia, on diazoxide	8 years
NC /M	Retardation	40 months	Normoglycemia and free of convulsions under diazoxide and anticonvulsants	Discharge from hospital

After the end of insulin dependence, four children exhibited normal serum glucose levels. Recurrent hypoglycemia was corrected by increasing carbohydrate intake in three cases and required temporary diazoxide medication in another four. In contrast to the preoperative course, diazoxide was successful in three cases and failed in one. In this child, however, serum glucose levels normalized spontaneously after a few months. The longest diazoxide dependence (12 months) was in a child who had undergone resection of only four-fifths of the pancreas. Pancreatectomy was unsuccessful in a boy already heavily retarded prior to surgery at 31 months of age who suffered from severe, recurrent hypoglycemia up to his 7th year, despite diazoxide medication.

The long-term results correlate closely with preoperative conditions as far as general development is concerned. Seven of eight children who were normally developed preoperatively showed age-corresponding development postoperatively as well. One child with slight retardation preoperatively made up for delayed development postoperatively. However, severe retardation and already manifest seizures did not improve by operation, even if serum glucose levels were normal after surgery (Table 2).

Discussion

The prime aim of long-term treatment of nesidioblastosis is the permanent and reliable prevention of hypoglycemia caused by hyperinsulinism. Only adequate therapy given in time can prevent development of retardation and cerebral convulsions [12].

The courses of disease in our patients as well as the experiences of other authors substantiate the fact that conservative treatment of nesidioblastosis with increased carbohydrate intake and diazoxide is ineffective or only temporarily effective in most cases. Accordingly, the long-term results of conservative treatment alone are unsatisfactory [10].

The importance of surgical therapy must be seen in this context. There can be no doubt that subtotal pancreatectomy is a risky, irreversible, and mutilating operation. We agree with other authors, however, that the surgical risk can be limited by a suitable surgical strategy and technique and is justified by favorable long-term results. With the reservation of a relatively short follow-up in two children, we had only one treatment failure; in this case, however, the conditions prior to surgery, at an age of 31 months and with severe preoperative retardation, were extremely poor. On the other hand, eight children developed normally following subtotal pancreatectomy, including those who required temporary diazoxide treatment postoperatively.

Our experience indicates that surgery should be performed as soon as the diagnosis is established. Pre-existing brain damage and convulsions cannot be cured by surgery, of course [4].

While preserving the common bile duct, pancreatic resection must be as nearly total as technically possible. The pancreatic remnant in the duodenal C-sling should be as small as feasible, but should render a secure closure of the stump. In our opinion, primary total pancreatectomy is not indicated. Considering the favorable results of subtotal pancreatectomy, a permanent, insulin-dependent diabetes is not justifiable a priori. Only in cases where normalization of glucose metabolism cannot be achieved by subtotal resection or by medical therapy may total pancreatectomy be indicated as the ultima ratio [6, 11].

References

1. Aynsly-Green A, Polak JM, Bloom SR, Gough MH, Keeling J, Ashcroft SJH, Turner RC, Baum JD (1981) Nesidioblastosis of the pancreas: definition of the syndrome and the management of the severe neonatal hyperinsulinaemic hypoglycaemia. Arch Dis Child 56:496–508
2. Bremer HJ (1983) Metabolisch bedingte Notfallsituationen des Neugeborenen. Monatsschr Kinderheilkd 131:317–320
3. Carcassone M, De Larue A, Le Tourneau JN (1983) Surgical treatment of organic pancreatic hypoglycemia in the pediatric age. J Pediatr Surg 18:75–79
4. Haberland R, Willberg B, Holschneider AM, Engelskirchen R, Gharib M (1988) Chirurgie des endokrinen Pankreas. Z Kinderchir 43:273–280
5. Laidlaw GF (1938) Nesidioblastoma, the islet tumor of the pancreas. Am J Pathol 14:125–134
6. Martin LW, Ryckman FC, Sheldon CA (1984) Experience with 95% pancreatectomy and splenic salvage for neonatal nesidioblastosis. Ann Surg 200:355–362
7. Müller E (1985) 14. International. Symposium der Österreichischen Gesellschaft für Kinderchirurgie. Obergurgl, 28–30 January
8. Rahier J, Fält K, Müntefering H, Becker K, Gepts W, Falkmer S (1984) The basic structural lesion of the persistent neonatal hypoglycaemia with hyperinsulinism: deficiency of pancreatic D cells or hyperactivity of B cells? Diabetologia 26:282–289
9. Saul W, Willberg B, Bremer HJ (1984) Die chirurgische Therapie der Nesidioblastose. Z Kinderchir 39:96–98
10. Schiller M, Krausz M, Meyer S, Lijovetzky G, Landau H (1980) Neonatal hyperinsulinismus – surgical and pathologic considerations. J Pediatr Surg 15:16–20
11. Simmons PS, Telander RL, Carney JA, Wold JE, Haymond MW (1984) Surgical management of hyperinsulinemic hypoglycemia in children. Arch Surg 19:520–525
12. Wendel U, Kardorff C, Dorittke P, Bremer HJ (1985) Somatostatin zur Notfallbehandlung bei persistierenden Hypoglykämien aufgrund eines Hyperinsulinismus (Nesidioblastose des Pankreas). Monatsschr Kinderheilkd 133:527–531

Surgical Treatment of Nesidioblastosis in Childhood

J. Dobroschke[1], R. Linder[2], and A. Otten[3]

Summary

A review of the literature on the surgical treatment of nesidioblastosis in childhood was made to answer the following questions: age at operation, surgical procedure, pathohistological findings, incidence of recurrence and its treatment, as well as mortality. Primary subtotal pancreatectomy appears to be the method of choice. It should be performed as early as possible following exact diagnosis. Total pancreatectomy is reserved for treatment of a recurrence.

Zusammenfassung

Eine Literaturübersicht zur chirurgischen Behandlung der kindlichen Nesidioblastose sollte Klarheit zu folgenden Fragen schaffen: Alter bei Operation, Operationstechnik, pathohistologische Befunde, Häufigkeit und Behandlung von Rezidiven und Letalität. Als Methode der Wahl beim Ersteingriff wird die subtotale Pankreatektomie angesehen. Diese soll nach exakter Diagnostik so früh wie möglich erfolgen. Die totale Pankreatektomie ist der Behandlung eines Rezidives vorbehalten.

Résumé

Une étude de la littérature sur le traitement chirurgical de la nésidioblastose des enfants devait répondre aux questions suivantes: âge lors de l'opération, technique chirurgicale, résultats histopathologiques, fréquence des récurrences, traitement et léthalité. Il en ressort que la pancréatectomie primaire subtotale est la méthode de choix. Elle doit être pratiquée aussitôt que possible après l'établissement du diagnostic. La pancréatectomie totale sera réservée au traitement d'une récurrence.

Introduction

The rareness of nesidioblastosis in childhood makes it difficult to report on its surgical treatment based on our own experience. It would be hard to find a general or pediatric surgeon who has personally handled more than a dozen such cases. Therefore, one is particularly dependent on the experience of other surgical teams

---

[1] Krankenhaus der Barmherzigen Brüder, Prüfeningerstraße 86, D-8400 Regensburg (W), FRG.
[2] Klinik für Allgemein- und Thoraxchirurgie am Zentrum für Chirurgie, Anästhesiologie und Urologie and
[3] Zentrum für Kinderheilkunde, Justus-Liebig-Universität Gießen, Klinikstraße 29, D-6300 Gießen (W), FRG.

Progress in Pediatric Surgery, Vol. 26
Gauderer and Angerpointner (Eds.)
© Springer-Verlag Berlin Heidelberg 1991

when choosing the best treatment in a given case. From the literature that has appeared in the past 5 years we have collected a group of comparable cases [1, 2, 4–11]. The important points were age at operation, surgical procedure, pathohistological findings, and incidence, treatment and mortality of recurrence.

Age at Operation

The decision to operate is made in close cooperation with a skilled pediatric endocrinologist. Likewise, the time of surgery should be fixed with the endocrinologist. Both the indication and the date for surgery are usually clear when the diagnosis has been made. In most instances this takes place within the first 2 months of life, at our institution in the third week (Table 1). Most infants who were operated on later had undergone examinations at other clinics for cerebro-organic diseases, similar to adult hyperinsulinism. If hypoglycemic states are recognized only after 1 year or later, one should consider a solitary adenoma in particular.

Surgical Procedure

The operation should be an elective procedure; emergency surgery is never necessary. A prerequisite to surgery is a balanced electrolyte metabolism; in particular, any hypokalemia must be under control. The acid-base relationship must be balanced and serum glucose levels should be within the normal range. Intraoperatively, these parameters should be closely monitored, since manipulation of the pancreas can increase insulin incretion and removal of pancreatic tissue can reduce it.

The aim of the operation is to reduce the endocrine potential of the pancreas. It ranges from the enucleation of a solitary adenoma, over a left-sided pancreatic resection with the removal of 75%–85% of the pancreatic tissue, to a subtotal pancreatectomy with a 85%–95% resection (Fig. 1). Solitary adenomas are extremely rare, especially in newborns. The possibility should be kept in mind in older children who present later with organic hyperinsulinism. Nevertheless, during surgery we first explore the pancreas carefully for possible nodules.

Table 1. Age at operation, based on a review of the literature covering 1981–1985 ($n = 51$)

Age at operation	No. of patients
Up to 2 months	28
2–6 months	13
6–12 months	4
Over 12 months	6

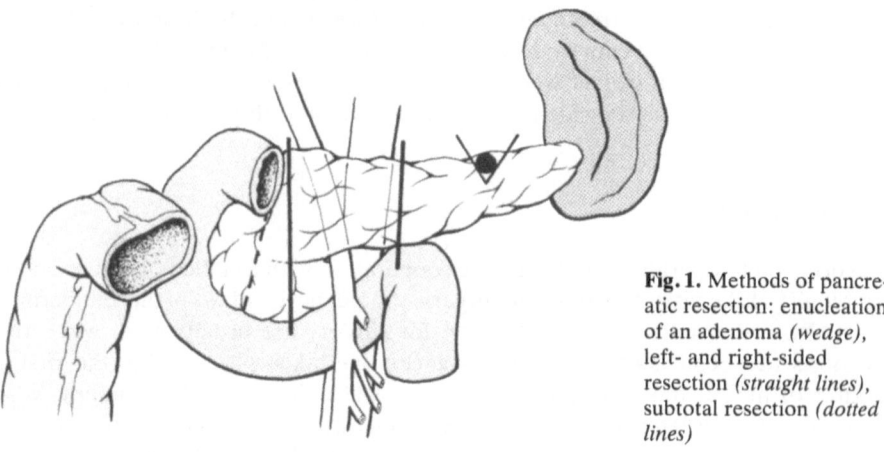

Fig. 1. Methods of pancreatic resection: enucleation
of an adenoma *(wedge)*,
left- and right-sided
resection *(straight lines)*,
subtotal resection *(dotted
lines)*

Table 2. Surgical procedures followed in 51 patients taken from the
literature 1981–1985

Procedure	No. of patients
Left-sided pancreatectomy (75%–85%)	36 (2 died)
Subtotal pancreatectomy (85%–95%)	14
Total pancreatectomy	–
Enucleation	1

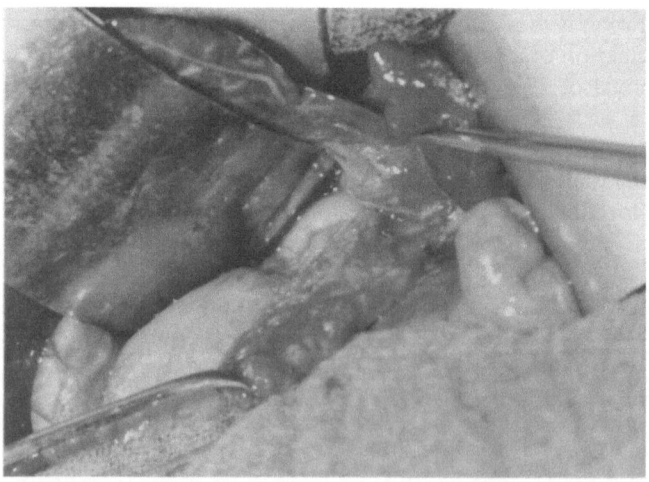

Fig. 2. Operative technique; mobilization of the pancreas with preservation of the spleen. Tail of
pancreas is lifted off and splenic vessels are dissected

In our opinion, primary total pancreatectomy is too radical. The problems of pancreoprivic diabetes are too high a price to pay for eliminating hyperinsulinism. A left-sided resection with removal of three quarters of the gland or a subtotal pancreatectomy should be carried out instead. Sometimes the term "near total pancreatectomy" appears in the literature. We consider this differentiation between subtotal and nearly total pancreatectomy merely academic. In any case, the resection plane is on the right side of the vessel axis. The amount of glandular tissue that remains should be just enough to make a secure closure of the resection area possible. We regard this subtotal pancreatectomy as the method of choice in the surgical treatment of nesidioblastosis in childhood.

Remarkably, the literature review revealed that only a left-sided pancreatic resection had been performed in the majority of cases, a subtotal pancreatectomy

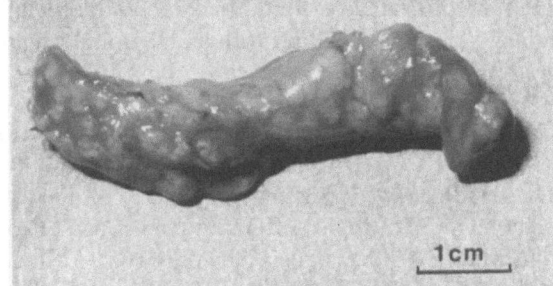

Fig. 3. Resection specimen after subtotal pancreatectomy (cm)

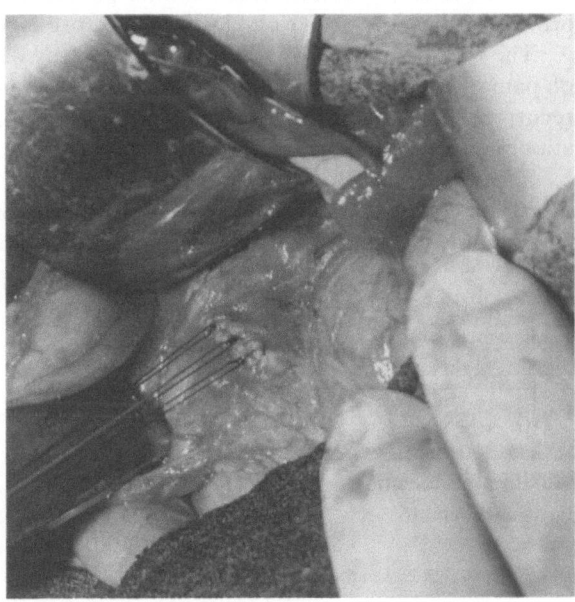

Fig. 4. Following subtotal pancreatic resection the resection plane is closed with interrupted sutures

in only 14 children. An enucleation was carried out once. Total pancreatectomy was never the primary therapeutic step (Table 2).

Technically, we start to mobilize the gland from the left; it is imperative that the spleen be preserved, in view of the danger of postsplenectomy sepsis (see Fig. 2). Dissection of the spenic vessels from the pancreas is easier in children than in adults. The resection should extend beyond the vessel axis to the right in any case (Fig. 3). The resection plane is closed by means of interrupted sutures (Fig. 4). We were not able to isolate the pancreatic duct for separate purse-string sutures in any of our three patients.

Pathohistological Findings

Histological examinations revealed predominantly multifocal proliferation. Isolated adenomas were found in three children, all over 1 year of age. Multifocal proliferation concomitant with an adenoma was reported in two cases (Table 3).

Late Results: Incidence of Recurrence, Its Treatment and Mortality

The incidence of recurrence in the 51 children who were operated on is surprisingly high: 30 of them suffered a recurrence (Table 4). The incidence was highest following left-sided pancreatectomy (67%), but 42% following subtotal pancreatectomy is also a depressing rate. This underlines the fact that left-sided pancreatectomy with 75%–85% resection is unsufficient and calls for the excision of as much tissue as possible during subtotal pancreatectomy. Total pancreatectomy, however, does not seem to be justified as a primary operation.

The question arises whether the recurrences were due to insufficient excision of pancreatic tissue or to real regeneration, as is sometimes described. If the recurrence appears only a few weeks following the operation, pancreatic regeneration must be assumed.

Ten of the patients with recurrences were conservatively treated with diazoxide. Subtotal pancreatectomy was carried out seven times and total pancreatectomy ten times. For the other three cases the treatment of recurrence is not

Table 3. Results of histological examination in 51 cases in the literature 1981–1985

Findings	No. of patients
Multifocal proliferation	46
Focal adenomatosis	–
Adenoma	3
Multifocal proliferation plus adenoma	2

Table 4. Incidence of recurrence following surgery for nesidioblastosis in 51 children (review of literature 1981–1985)

Primary surgical procedure	No. of recurrences (%)
Left-sided pancreatectomy (75%–85%)	24/36 (67)
Subtotal pancreatectomy (85%–95%)	6/14 (42)
Enucleation	0/ 1 (0)
Total	30/51 (59)

Table 5. Treatment of 30 reccurences

Treatment method	No. of patients
Conservative	10 (2 died)
Subtotal pancreatectomy	7
Total pancreatectomy	10 (1 died)
Not reported	3

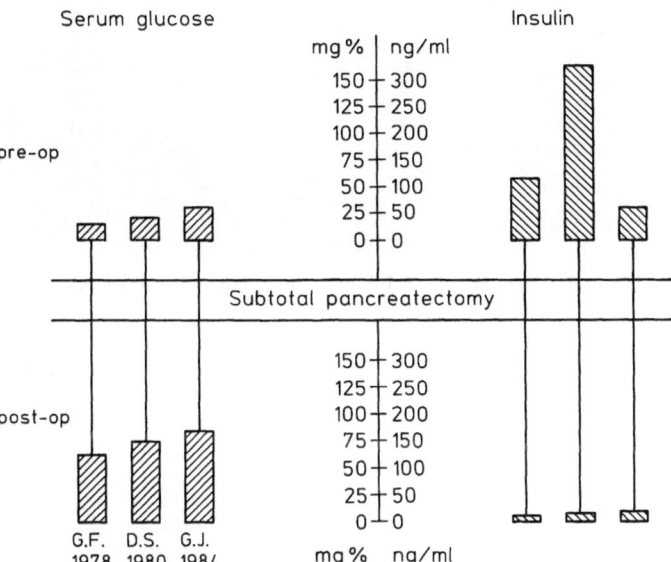

Fig. 5. Pre- and postoperative levels of serum glucose and insulin in three children with nesidioblastosis treated at the Surgical Clinic of the University of Gießen

reported. Total pancreatectomy seems to be the method of choice in the treatment of recurrences (Table 5).

We have operated on three children for nesidioblastosis. All presented preoperatively with extremely low serum glucose levels which required i.v. glucose substitution. Corresponding insulin levels were very high. Subtotal pancreatectomy was carried immediately after the diagnosis was established. Postoperatively, serum glucose, insulin and C-peptide levels normalized (Fig. 5). All children are free of recurrence 8, 6 and 2 years, respectively, after surgery. Their development has been normal without insulin substitution. Only during the first 6 postoperative months was substitution with exocrine pancreatic enzymes necessary.

By means of collagenase digestion, microfragments of Langerhans islets were extracted from the resection specimen of the child who was operated (Fig. 6).

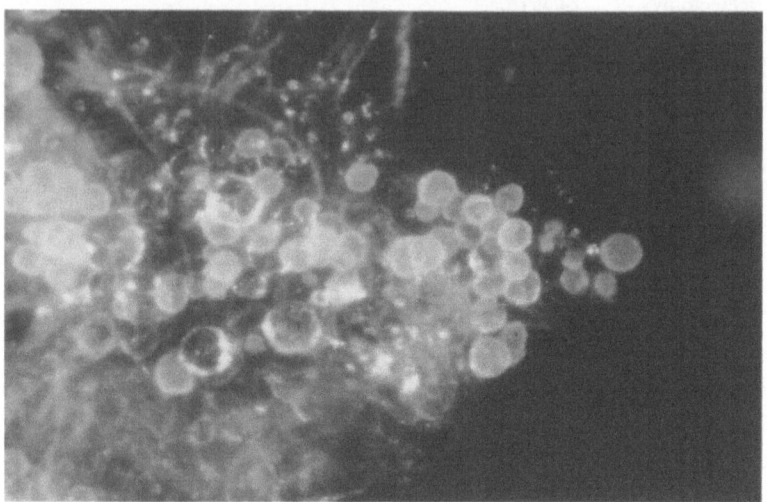

Fig. 6. Microfragments of Langerhans inslets extracted from a resection specimen by means of collagenase digestion

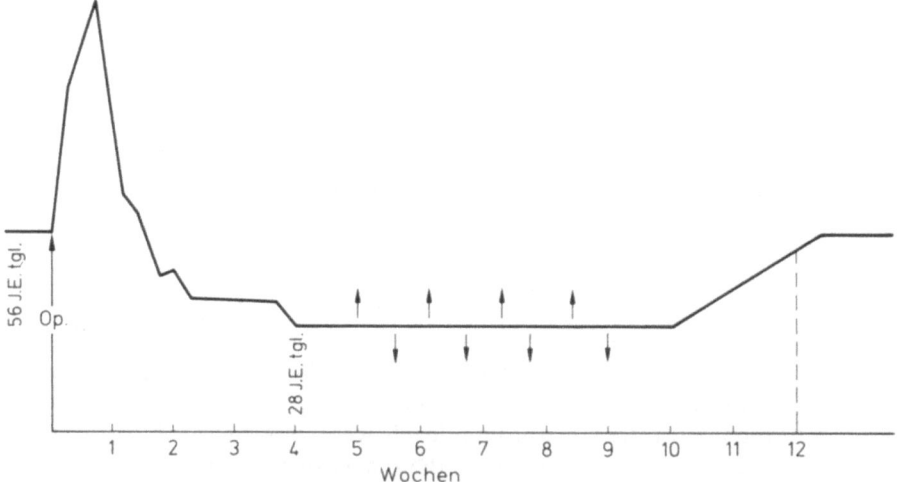

Fig. 7. Insulin requirement of a 45-year-old diabetic prior to and following islet cell transplantation. *J. E. tgl*, IU daily

These were injected for treatment of diabetes into the spleen of a 45-year-old diabetic patient who had undergone kidney transplantation 4 weeks earlier [3]. Four weeks later, at least a partial effect of the transplant was seen. For a further 6 weeks, this patient required only half of the insulin dose which had been necessary preoperatively (Fig. 7). However, his insulin requirement increased again thereafter. The transplanted Langerhans islets fell victim to either rejection or fibrosis.

To summarize, it can be stated that subtotal pancreatectomy is the method of choice for treatment of nesidioblastosis in childhood. The operation should be carried out as soon as possible after establishment of the diagnosis. Total pancreatectomy should be reserved for the treatment of recurrence.

References

1. Aynsley-Green A, Polak JM, Bloom SR, Gouch MH, Keeling J, Ashcroft SJH, Turner RC, Baum JD (1981) Nesidioblastosis of the pancreas: definition of the syndrome and the management of the severe neonatal hyperinsulinaemic hypoglycaemia. Arch Dis Child 56:496–508
2. Bindewald H, Heinze E, Merkle P (1982) Chirurgische Therapie der Nesidioblastosis im Kindesalter. Langenbecks Arch Chir 356:299–302
3. Dobroschke J, Schwemmle K, Langhoff G, Bretzel RG (1983) Allotransplantation of neonatal pancreas-microfragments in man. Horm Metab Res [Suppl] 13:91–93
4. Gough MH (1984) The surgical treatment of hyperinsulinism in infancy and childhood. Br J Surg 71:75–78
5. Jeschke R, Romen W, Thanner F, Niggemeyer H (1978) Zum Krankheitsbild der diffusen, nesidioblastischen Inselhyperplasie im Neugeborenen- und Säuglingsalter. Klin Padiatr 191:403–411
6. Kramer JL, Bell MJ, DeSchryver K, Bower RJ, Ternberg JL, White NH (1981) Clinical and histologic indications for extensive pancreatic resection in nesidioblastosis. AQm J Surg 143:116–119
7. Landau H, Perlman M, Meyer S, Isacsohn M, Krausz M, Mayan H, Lijovetzky G, Schiller M (1982) Persistent neonatal hypoglycemia due to hyperinsulinism: medical aspects. Pediatrics 70:440–446
8. Lloyd RV, Caceres V, Warner TFCS, Gilbert EF (1981) Islet cell adenomatosis. A report of two cases and review of the literature. Arch Pathol Lab Med 105:198–202
9. Moazam F, Rodgers BM, Talbert JL, Rosenbloom AL (1982) Near-total pancreatectomy in persistent infantile hypoglycemia. Arch Surg 117:1151–1154
10. Rahier J, Fält K, Müntefering H, Becker K, Gepts W, Falkmer S (1984) The basic structural lesion of persistent neonatal hypoglycaemia with hyperinsulinism: deficiency of pancreatic D cells or hyperactivity of B cells? Diabetologia 26:282–289
11. Töpke B, Menzel K, Kasper JM (1985) Nesidioblastose − eine seltene Ursache kongenitaler persistierender Hyperglykämien. Kinderarztl Prax 53:291–295

Total Pancreatectomy in a Case of Nesidioblastosis Due to Persisting Hyperinsulinism Following Subtotal Pancreatectomy

P. Dohrmann, W. Mengel, and J. Splieth

Summary

Hypoglycemia with hyperinsulinism persisted in a newborn weighing 6410 g despite treatment with high doses of diazoxide and glucagon, as well as infusions of glucose and somatostatin. A subtotal pancreatectomy was performed after nesidioblastosis had been diagnosed on the basis of the laboratory findings. Due to the persistence of therapy-resistant hypogycemia, a total pancreatectomy preserving the duodenum and the bile duct was done 6 weeks later. With insulin and pancreatic enzyme substitution the now 6-year, 9-month-old child has shown normal, age, appropriate development.

Zusammenfassung

Bei einem 6410 g schweren Neugeborenen persistierte eine Hypoglykämie mit Hyperinsulinismus trotz hochdosierter Diazoxid- und Glukagonbehandlung sowie Glukoseinfusionen und Somatostatininfusion. Nachdem laborchemisch die Diagnose einer Nesidioblastose gestellt wurde, erfolgte primär die subtotale Pankreasresektion. Bei anhaltenden therapieresistenten Hypoglykämien erfolgte 6 Wochen später die totale Pankreatektomie unter Erhaltung des Duodenums und des Ductus choledochus. Das nunmehr 6¾ Jahre alte Kind hat sich unter Insulin- und Pankreonsubstitution altersentsprechend normal entwickelt.

Résumé

Chez un nouveau-né pesant 6410 g, on constatait une hypoglycémie persistante et une hyperinsulinie en dépit de l'administration à hautes doses de diazoxide et de glucagon et de perfusions de glucose et de somatostatine. Les résultats de l'examen en laboratoire ayant confirmé le diagnostic de nésidioblastose, l'enfant subit d'abord une pancréatectomie subtotale puis, six semaines plus tard, une pancréatectomie totale, conservant le duodénum et le canal cholédoque car l'hypoglycémie résistait au traitement. Cet enfant, qui a maintenant 6 ans et 9 mois, est traité avec une substitution d'insuline et de pancréatine, et sa croissance et son développement sont normaux pour son âge.

Introduction

Nesidioblastosis is characterized by the persistence of early fetal islet cell formation from pluripotent cells, which leads to hyperinsulinism. This involves a pro-

Department of General Surgery, Pediatric Surgery, Arnold-Heller Straße 7, D-2300 Kiel 1 (W), FRG.

Progress in Pediatric Surgery, Vol. 26
Gauderer and Angerpointner (Eds.)
© Springer-Verlag Berlin Heidelberg 1991

nounced proliferation of B cells which are spread diffusely over the entire pancreas [2, 5, 7]. A clinical sign during the first days of life is severe hypoglycemia that can hardly be influenced by drugs. This results in an increased spasmophilia, which causes infantile brain damage if treated inadequately.

Persisting uncontrollable hypoglycemia and demonstrated hyperinsulinism are indications for surgical intervention. A subtotal pancreatectomy preserving only a narrow pancreatic rest on the duodenal C is the procedure of choice. In a case of persisting resistance to therapy a total pancreatectomy is necessary, and when performing this operation it is possible to preserve the duodenum and the choledochus. Based on a case of ours, these aspects are presented and reported in the following.

Case Report

The little girl we treated is the second child of a healthy mother. The infant, delivered by cesarean section, had a birth weight of 6410 g and measured 60 cm in length (Fig. 1). Pronounced adiposity and hypertrichosis were evident; the infant also suffered from cardiac insufficiency. Apnea and a convulsive fit with a blood-sugar value below 10 mg/dl occurred shortly after delivery. The further development was characterized by therapy-resistant hypoglycemia which persisted despite glucose infusion rates of up to 10 mg/kg body wt./min and the additional administration of prednisone and diazoxide. Since the laboratory findings (insulin-glucose quotient, lacking suppression of insulin in the epinephrine test, somatostatin test) were indicative of nesidioblastosis, surgery was decided upon at the age of 6 weeks.

A subtotal pancreatectomy was performed at first, leaving only an extremely narrow parenchymal rest in the duodenal C. The postoperative course was uncomplicated. After initial, short-term attacks of hyperglycemia, the condition developed once again on the 10th day. The maximum utilization of conservative treatment was unsuccessful; even high doses of somatostatin did not satisfactorily control the hypoglycemia. Thus, it proved necessary to perform a relaparotomy and to remove the remaining parenchyma as in a total pancreatectomy. It was possible to resect the remaining pancreatic tissue while preserving the duodenum and the bile duct. The postoperative course once again was uncomplicated. As had been expected, diabetes mellitus developed, requiring a daily insulin dose of 0.2 units/kg.

The histological findings confirmed the nesidioblastosis, with a pronounced multiplication of the B cells, an islet cell proliferation from epithelial cells along the efferent ducts, and a slight polymorphism and hypochromasia of the nuclei. During the further development the cardiac insufficiency returned to normal and both adiposity and hirsutism regressed. Convulsive fits were no longer observed.

By now, the patient is 6 years and 9 months of age (Fig. 2)and has had regular check-ups. The child receives pancreatic enzymes and insulin, and her somatic-psychosomatic development is normal.

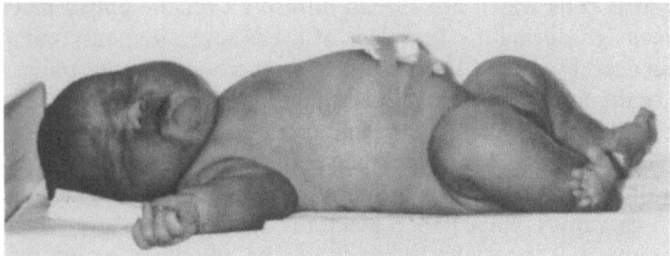

Fig. 1. A newborn with nesidioblastosis weighing 6410 g

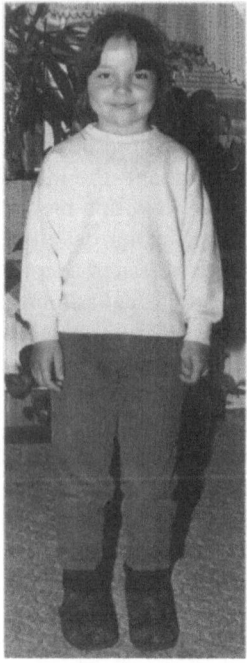

Fig. 2. The same child at 6 years and 9 months after total pancreatectomy

Discussion

If nesidioblastosis is diagnosed in a newborn, and if it proves resistant to conservative treatment, immediate surgical intervention is indicated. There is a high risk of irreversible brain damage if surgery is delayed [8]. It is for this reason that early subtotal pancreatectomy is well established as a method of primary surgical treatment. It should be directed to right above the mesenteric vessels, leaving only a narrow parenchymal edge [1, 9].

Goudswaad et al. [3] call for a "near-total pancreatectomy" if therapy-resistent hypoglycemia should occur once more. In cases of persistent hypoglycemia following subtotal pancreatectomy, Harken et al. [4] report a total pancreatectomy to be very successful, as does the Bern University Hospital, where 11 patients were treated by this method [10].

Thomas et al. [8] and Morger [6] succeeded in preserving the choledochus and the duodenum when performing the necessary pancreatectomy. With persisting hypoglycemia after subtotal pancreatectomy a relaparotomy initially was undertaken with hesitation, and only after every possibility of conservative treatment had been exhausted. Nowadays, immediate total pancreatectomy is being demanded more and more [3] in order to avoid the danger of brain damage.

Our results with a follow-up period of 6 and ¾ years are encouraging and support this conclusion. The risk of mental retardation was avoided. The diabetes mellitus can be controlled without any problems by administration of insulin. As yet, no malabsorption syndrome has been diagnosed. The development of the little girl is normal and appropriate for her age; she has no problems in meeting the prescholastic standards.

References

1. Dobroschke J, Linder R, Otten A (1986) Chirurgische Behandlung der kindlichen Nesidioblastose. Arbeitsgemeinschaft Chirurgische Endokrinologie 5th Symposium, 19–20 Sept, Hamburg
2. Dutrillaux MC, Hollande E, Rozé C (1979) Occurrence and cytodifferentiation of mucopolysaccharide-secreting cells in the pancreas of children with nesidioblastosis. Virchows Arch [B] 30:195–208
3. Goudswaard WB, Zwiestra RP, Houthoff HJ, Rouwe C, Kootstra G (1984) Surgical treatment of organic hyperinsulinism in infancy. Surgical procedure in the absence of a demonstrable insulinoma and a peroperative diagnosis of nesidioblastosis. Z Kinderchir 39:91–95
4. Harken AH, Filler RM, AvRuskin TW, Crigler JF (1971) The role of "total" pancreatectomy in the treatment of unremitting hypoglycemia of infancy. J Pediatr Surg 6:284–289
5. Klöppel G (1981) Spezielle pathologische Anatomie. Pathologie der endokrinen Organe. Springer, Berlin Heidelberg New York, pp 618–728
6. Morger R (1983) Surgical operations on pancreas in malignant disease in children. In: Rickham PP, Hecker WCh, Prévot J (eds) Progress in pediatric surgery. Endocrine disorders and tumors in children, vol 16. Urban & Schwarzenberg, Baltimore, pp 63–70
7. Schwarz SS, Rich BH, Lucky AW, Straus FH, Gonen B, Wolfsdorf J, Thorb FW, Burrington JD, Madden JD, Rubenstein A, Rosenfield AH (1979) Familial nesidioblastosis: severe neonatal hypoglycemia in two families. J Pediatr 95:44–53
8. Thomas CG, Underwood LE, Carney CN, Dolcourt JL, Whitt JJ (1977) Neonatal and infantile hypoglycemia due to insulin excess: new aspects of diagnosis and surgical management. Ann Surg 185:506–517
9. Willberg B (1986) Kindliche Nesidioblastose – Chirurgische Therapie. Arbeitsgemeinschaft Chirurgische Endokrinologie 5th Symposium, 19–20 Sept, Hamburg
10. Zuppinger K (1983) Disorders of the endocrine pancreas. In: Rickham PP, Hecker WCh, Prévot J (eds) Progress in pediatric surgery. Endocrine disorders and tumors in children, vol 16. Urban and Schwarzenberg, Baltimore, pp 51–61

Pancreatic Head Tumor in a Child

C. Deindl

Summary

A 13-year-old girl with pancreatic head tumor required a pancreatoduodenectomy (Whipple procedure). Pathohistological examination disclosed a pancreatic apudoma. The characteristics of this very rare tumor, its symptoms and treatment are described.

Zusammenfassung

Es wird über ein 13jähriges Mädchen mit einem Pankreaskopftumor berichtet, der eine Duodenopankreatektomie (Whipple-Operation) erforderlich machte. Die pathohistologische Untersuchung ergab ein Apudom des Pankreas. Die Charakteristika dieses sehr seltenen Tumors sowie Symptome und Behandlung werden beschrieben.

Résumé

Une fillette de 13 ans présentant une tumeur de la tête du pancréas a subi une pancréatectomie et duodénectomie associée (opération de Whipple). L'examen histopathologique révéla un apudome pancréatique. Les caractéristiques de cette tumeur extrêmement rare, les symptômes et le traitement sont décrits.

A 13-year-old girl with an uneventful history was transfered to our institution in February 1984 with a palpable mass extending from the epigastrium to the umbilicus. A plain abdominal X-ray disclosed an extended tumor in the upper right and middle abdomen. Abdominal ultrasound revealed a solid tumor with an inhomogeneous echostructure and calcifications measuring $15 \times 12 \times 7$ cm and originating from the pancreatic area. The right kidney, liver and great abdominal vessels were free. On laparotomy, a pancreatic head tumor with irregular surface, infiltrating the mesenterium and the ascending colon, was found; it was easily mobilized. Macroscopically, the tumor appeared to be malignant; hence, a duodenopancreatectomy (Whipple procedure) was carried out. Figures 1 and 2 show the pre- and postoperative situs. Pathohistological examination showed the tumor to extend to the duodenum, 3 cm distal to the pylorus, with ulceration of the

Pediatric Surgical Clinic (Dir. Prof. Dr. I. Joppich), Dr. von Haunersches Kinderspital of the University of Munich, Lindwurmstraße 4, D-8000 Munich 2 (W), FRG.

Progress in Pediatric Surgery, Vol. 26
Gauderer and Angerpointner (Eds.)
© Springer-Verlag Berlin Heidelberg 1991

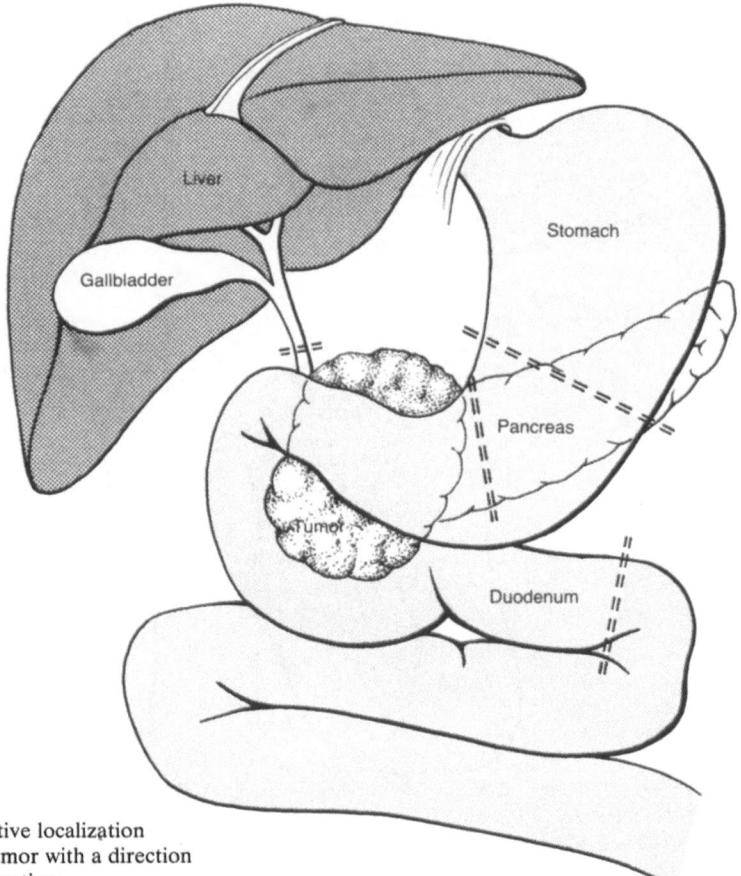

Fig. 1. Intraoperative localization
of the pancreas tumor with a direction
for the area of resection

duodenal wall. The common bile duct was not involved and resection borders
were tumor free. Microscopically, tumor nodules with follicular structure but
without cell atypia or mitosis were found (Fig. 3). The edges of the tumor contained normal exocrine pancreatic tissue and a pseudocapsule. A destructive infiltration of surrounding tissues was not shown.

Immunohistological investigations disclosed a faint antibody reaction against
somatostatin, the tumor thus representing a somatostatinoma. Somatostatinomas
typically do not cause clinical symptoms [19]. Immunohistological reactions with
gastrin, serotonin, pancreatic polypeptides, insulin and glucagon were negative.
Electron microscopy revealed numerous intracellular granules.

Thus, this endocrine pancreatic head tumor was a so-called pancreatic
apudoma, or carcinoid [11, 20]. The origin of the tumor is the APUD cells (amine
precursor uptake and decarboxylation cells), first described by Pearse in 1968
[21]. Apudomas are very rare, with a postmortem incidence under 1% [10]. There

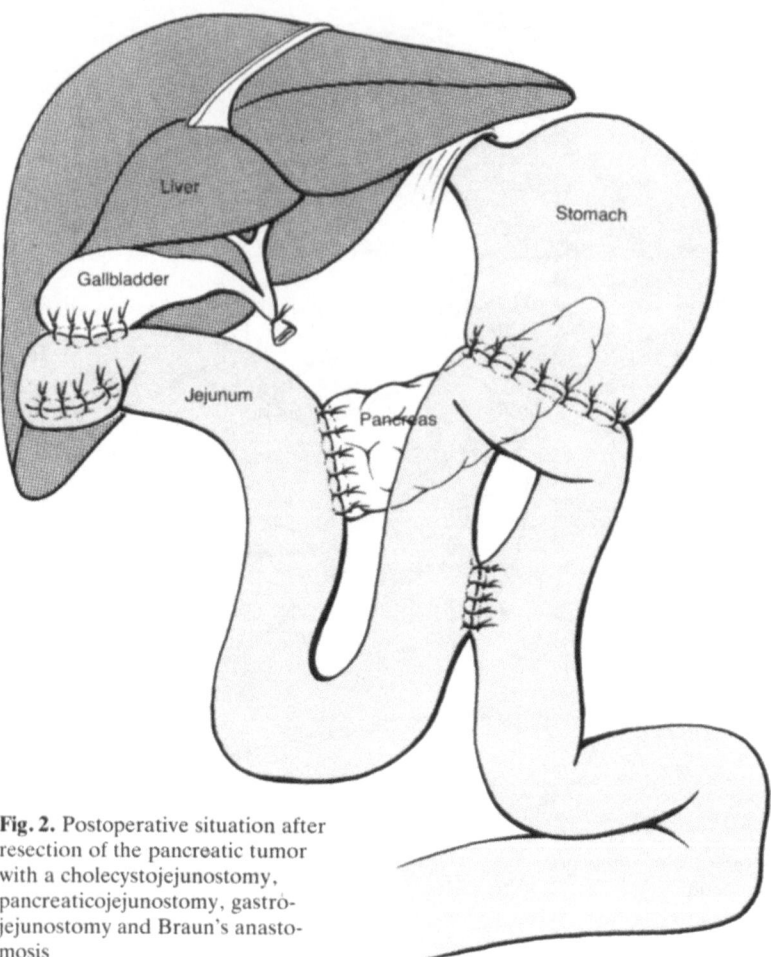

Fig. 2. Postoperative situation after resection of the pancreatic tumor with a cholecystojejunostomy, pancreaticojejunostomy, gastrojejunostomy and Braun's anastomosis

is considerable variation of tumor localization, for instance in the central nervous system, bronchial system, gastrointestinal tract, (para)thyroid gland, placenta and adrenal glands [14, 21]. A search of the literature [7, 21, 22, 25, 30] revealed that only one apudoma in a child had been described so far [9]. Pancreatic tumors are generally rare in children [17, 29]. The origin of an endocrine pancreatic tumor is almost invariably an islet cell [1, 2, 4, 10, 27, 28]. These tumors can also occur within the framework of a MEN (*M*ultiple *E*ndorince *N*eoplasia) syndrome, or with the Sipple or Werner syndromes [26]. There is a difference between endocrine active and inactive tumors [16, 27]. From 1967 to 1976, nearly 300 patients in West Germany were operated on for endocrine pancreatic tumors, 30% of which were endocrine inactive [18].

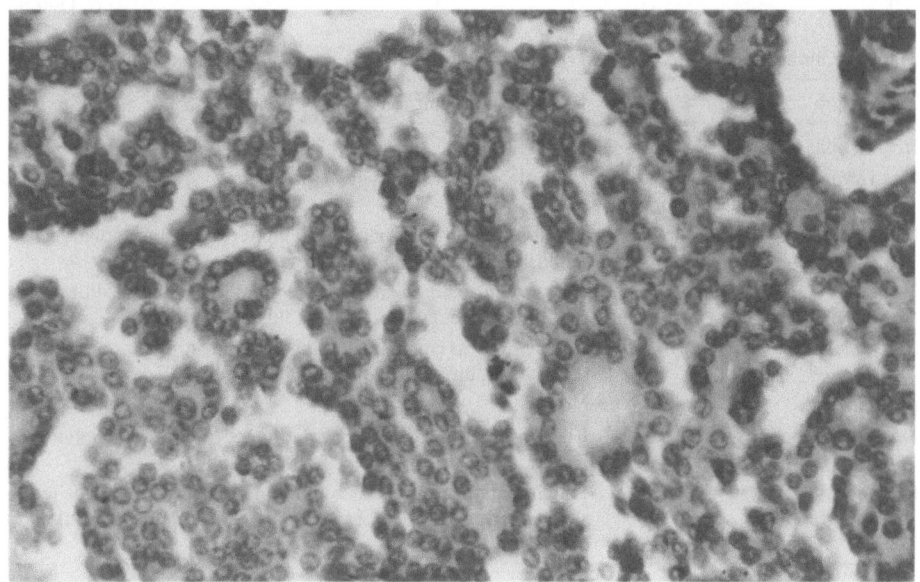

Fig. 3. Resection specimen showing tumor nodules with follicular structure but no cell atypia or mitosis. PAS, × 210

Table 1. Endocrine tumors of the pancreas and gastrointestinal tract [19]

Name	Cells	Hormone	Localization	Proportion of tumors malignant (%)	Multiple endocrine neoplasia (%)
Insulinoma	B	Insulin	Pancreas	5	5
Gastinoma	G	Gastrin, pancreatic polypeptide	Pancreas, duodenum, stomach	60–80	25
Glucagonoma	A	Glucagon	Pancreas	60	5
Vipoma		Vasoactive intestinal peptide (neurotensin) (peptide, histidine), isoleucine	Pancreas, extra-pancreatic ganglioneuro-blastoma	50	5
Somatostatinoma	D	Somatostatin	Pancreas, small bowel	90	5
pp-oma	pp	Pancreatic peptide	Pancreas	75	15
Neurotensinoma	NT	Neurotensin Vasoactive poly-peptide	Pancreas Sympathetic nervous system	50	10
Carcinoid	EC	Serotonin Kallikrein	Appendix Small bowel and colon, stomach, lung	Appendix under 3, other locali-zations nearly 30	10

Table 2. Clinical symptoms of endocrine-active tumors of the gastrointestinal tract [19]

Tumor	Typical clinic symptoms
Insulinoma	Hypoglycemia
Gastrinoma (Zollinger-Ellison syndrome)	Multiple ulcers with atypical localization
Glucagonoma	Exanthema, atrophic glossitis, venous thrombosis, diabetes mellitus, anemia, weight loss, diarrhea
Vipoma (Verner-Morrison syndrome)	Heavy watery diarrhea, hypokalemia, muscular weakness, renal insufficiency, weight loss, flush, achlorhydria
Somatostatinoma	Few symptoms (incident finding by laparotomy); sometimes diabetes mellitus, steatorrhea, cholecystolithiasis
pp-oma	No specific symptoms
Neurotensinoma	Like vipoma (because often simultaneous with vasoactive intestinal peptide)
Carcinoid	Hepatic metastases and carcinoid of lung and ovary: flushed skin, diarrhea, bronchial spasm, endocardial fibrosis of the right heart

Table 1 shows a classification of endocrine tumors of the pancreas and the gastrointestinal tract. Almost all of them can affect the pancreas, and their malignant potential is very high. Typical symptoms are described in Table 2. Leading symptoms of pancreatic tumors are abdominal pain, palpable mass, or obstruction of the common bile duct with jaundice [9, 23]. In cases with endocrine-active tumors, recurrent hypoglycemia, peptic ulcers, and the so-called carcinoid syndrome may appear (flush, diarrhea, fibrosis of the cardiac valves, skin involvement such as pellagra, bronchial obstruction, depression) [5, 6, 8, 22, 26, 27]. The first diagnostic tool is abdominal ultrasound, followed by CT, ERCP, and selective angiography [27]. Sometimes the serum levels of lipase, amylase, leucine amino-peptidase, or arginine carboxy peptidase are elevated. In our patient all these parameters were normal. Prognosis depends chiefly on whether the endocrine pancreatic tumor is malignant or benign. Not only morphological criteria but also the ability to develop metastases is a secure parameter of the tumor's malignant or benign nature [22]. The incidence of malignancies ranges from 5% for insulinomas to over 60% for gastrinomas [22]. Late metastases up to 19 years after first manifestation of the primary tumor have been described [10]. Therefore, long-term follow-up is mandatory.

High serum levels of alpha-HCG can be expected with 85% of malignant tumors [12], so the normal levels of alpha-HCG in our patient constituted a sign of benignity. The girl is now 18 years old and in good condition without signs of metastases or tumor relapse.

The treatment of choice for pancreatic tumors is surgical excision, since malignant pancreatic tumors are often insensitive to chemotherapy or irradiation. Operative procedures are tumor enucleation, partial pancreatic resection, or pancreatoduodenectomy (Whipple's operation), as was performed in our case

[1, 3, 9, 10, 13, 23, 24]. In patients with inoperable tumors treatment with streptomycin or 5-fluorouracil is recommended [15, 22].

References

1. Bedacht R, Rueff FL (1968) Insulinproduzierende und nicht-insulinproduzierende Pankreastumoren mit endokrinen Krankheitsbildern. Munch Med Wochenschr 8:446–454
2. Berk JE, Haubrich WS (1966) Tumors of the pancreas. In: Bockus HL (ed) Gastroenterology, 2nd edn. vol 2 Saunders, Philadelphia, pp 1021–1051
3. Bienayme J, Gross P (1976) Tumeurs malignes du pancreas chez l'enfant. Ann Chir Infant 17:131
4. Bloodwerth JMB Jr (1982) Endocrine pathology: general and surgical, 2nd edn. 1. Digestive and respiratory system. Williams and Wilkins, Baltimore, pp 531–555
5. Cassidy MA (1930) Abdominal carcinomatosis with probable adrenal involvement. Proc R Soc Med 24:139
6. Creutzfeldt W, Frerichs H, Ketterer H, Feurle G, Arnold R (1971) Klinische Syndrome hormonal aktiver Pankreastumoren: Diagnose und Differentialdiagnose. Chirurg 12:97–105
7. Grybosky J, Walker WA (1983) Tumors of the pancreas. In: Grybosky J (ed) Gastroenterologic problems in the infant, 2nd edn. Saunders, Philadelphia, pp 419–423
8. Hall TC (1974) Ectopic synthesis and paraneoplastic syndromes. Cancer 34:2088–2091
9. Hartmann G, Göring G (1968) Benignes Adenom des Pankreaskopfes bei einem Kind. Zentralbl Chir 93:1687–1692
10. Heidrich W, Kubale R, Seitz G, Weber T (1986) Endokriner Pancreastumor − Kasuistischer Beitrag zur Differentialdiagnostik zystischer Oberbauchtumoren. Ultraschall Med 7:138–140
11. Heitz PU (1984) Pancreatic endocrine tumors. In: Klöppel G, Heitz PU (eds) Pancreatic pathology. Churchill Livingstone, Edinburgh, pp 206–233
12. Heitz PU, Kaspar M, Klöppel G, Polak J, Vaitukaitis JL (1983) Glycoprotein-hormone alpha-chain production by pancreatic endocrine tumors: a specific marker for malignancy. Cancer 51:277–282
13. Jaubert de Beaujeu M, Chabal J, Metais B, Maurel C (1974) Duodenopancreatectomie céphalique pour tumeur pancreatique chez un enfant de 4 ans deni. Pediatrie 19:369–373
14. Johnson D (1981) Gastrointestinal endocrinology. In: Brook CDG (ed) Pediatric endocrinology. Blackwell, Oxford, pp 565–576
15. Kessinger A, Foley JF, Lemon HM (1983) Therapy of malignant APUD-cell tumors. Cancer 51:790–794
16. Klöppel G (1984) Pancreatic non-endocrine tumors. In: Klöppel G, Heitz PU (eds) Pancreatic pathology. Churchill Livingstone. Edinburgh, pp 79–114
17. Klöppel G, Held G, Marohoshi T, Seifert G (1982) Klassifikation exokriner Pankreastumoren. Pathologe 3:319–328
18. Kümmerle F, Rückert K (1978) Chirurgie des endokrinen Pankreas in der Bundesrepublik. Dtsch Med Wochenschr 13:729–733
19. Marbet UA, Kraenzlin M, Gyr K, Stalder GA (1986) Endokrin aktive Magen-Darm-Tumoren: Gibt es neue therapeutische Möglichkeiten? Dtsch Med Wochenschr 111:1120–1123
20. Oberndorfer S (1907) Karzinoide Tumoren des Dünndarmes. Z Pathol 1:426
21. Pearse AGE, Polak JM (1974) Endocrine tumors of neural chest origin: neurolophomas, apudomas and the APUD concept. Med Biol 53:13–18
22. Peiper H-J (1980) Pankreatische APUDome. Chirurg 51:380–383
23. Ravitch MM, Welch KJ, Benson CD, Aberdeen E, Randolph JG (eds) (1979) The pancreas: pancreas-neoplasm. Pediatric surgery, 3rd edn, vol 2. Yearbook Medical, Chicago, pp 865–868
24. Rickham PP (1975) Islet cell tumors in childhood. J Pediatr Surg 10:83–86
25. Ricour C, Duhamel JF, Lesee G, Schweisguth O (1977) Diarhee choleriforme dans un cas de ganglioneuroblastome. Arch Fr Pediatr 34:552–555

26. Röher HD, Branscheid D (1986) Multiple endokrine Neoplasien − MEN Typ I und II − in klinischer Erscheinung, diagnostischer und chirurgisch-therapeutischer Strategie. Chirurg 57:533−540
27. Rothmund M, Rückert K, Beyer J (1986) Insulinome und seltene endokrine Pankreastumoren. Chirurg 55:541−551
28. Silverman A, Roy CC (1983) Pancreastumor. In: Silverman A, Roy CC. Pediatric clinical gastroenterology, 3rd edn. Mosby, St. Louis, pp 490−493
29. Wilander E, Sundström C, Meurling S, Grotte G (1976) A highly differentiated exocrine pancreatic tumor in a young boy. Acta Paediatr Scand 65:769−772
30. Wood SM, Polak JM, Polak SR (1983) Gastrointestinal endocrine tumors. In: Hodgson HJ, Bloom SR, (eds) Gastrointestinal and hepatobiliary cancer. Chapman Hall, London, pp 207

Pheochromocytoma in Childhood

E. W. Fonkalsrud

Summary

Pheochromocytomas are uncommon tumors of childhood, accounting for 1% of hypertension cases in this age-group. Children have a high incidence of bilateral, multiple, or extra-adrenal tumors and a low incidence of malignancy. Alpha- and beta-blocking agents administered preoperatively have reduced complications markedly. Transabdominal resection is recommended because of the frequent extra-adrenal sites and multicentricity of the tumor in children. The mortality for removal of pheochromocytomas in childhood is currently less than 3%.

Zusammenfassung

Phäochromozytome sind bei Kindern seltene Tumoren und sind für nur 1% der Hypertoniefälle in dieser Altersgruppe verantwortlich. Bei Kindern liegen häufig bilaterale, multiple oder extraadrenale Tumoren vor, die zudem selten maligne sind. Präoperativ verabreichte α- und β-Blocker haben die Komplikationsrate beträchtlich gesenkt. Die transabdominelle Resektion wird empfohlen wegen der häufigen extraadrenalen Lokalisation und Multizentrizität bei Kindern. Die Operationsletalität des Phäochromozytoms im Kinderalter liegt derzeit unter 3%.

Résumé

Le phéochromocytome est une tumeur rare chez les enfants, responsable de 1% des cas d'hypertension à cet âge. Les enfants présentent un certain nombre de tumeurs bilatérales, multiples ou situées hors de la glande surrénale et peu de tumeurs malignes. L'administration d' alpha- et de bétabloquants avant l'opération réduit considérablement les complications. Il est recommandé de pratiquer une résection transabdominale car le siège est souvent hors de la glande surrénale et la tumeur, multifocale chez les enfants. La mortalité due à la résection des phéochromocytomes chez les enfants à l'heure actuelle de moins de 3%.

Introduction

Although Frankel [1], in 1886, reported the first case of a hypertensive syndrome with retinitis and bilateral adrenal tumors in an 18-year-old girl, it was not until 1922 that a clear relation between paroxysmal hypertension and adrenal medullary tumors was established by Labbe et al. [2]. In 1912, Pick [3] named the tumor for its predominant cell, the pheochromocyte.

Division of Pediatric Surgery, UCLA School of Medicine, Los Angeles, CA 90024, USA.

Progress in Pediatric Surgery, Vol. 26
Gauderer and Angerpointner (Eds.)
© Springer-Verlag Berlin Heidelberg 1991

Pheochromocytoma is a somewhat rare but important cause of correctable hypertension in children, as first observed by Kremer in 1936 [4]. This tumor is responsible for approximately 1% of the cases of childhood hypertension, typically occurring between the ages of 8 and 14 years. In 1963, Stackpole et al. [5] reported 100 cases of pheochromocytoma in children under the age of 14 years. Adults, on the other hand, have an overall incidence of pheochromocytoma estimated to be only one in 6000 hypertensive patients [6]. The right adrenal is involved approximately twice as often as the left. There is a slight preponderance of females, particularly in adolescence, which suggests that hormonal influences of puberty and growth may be etiologic factors. Whereas approximately 7% of pheochromocytomas are bilateral in adults, Hume [7] observed that 24% are bilateral in children. Others have noted the incidence of bilateral pheochromocytoma to be as high as 70% in children followed over the course of many years [8]. Extra-adrenal pheochromocytomas are present in approximately 30% of cases in children, about twice as common as in adults. They are most frequently found in the paraganglia, the organs of Zuckerkandl, and the bladder. Extra-abdominal tumors may develop in the brain, thorax, or neck [9].

Symptoms

The average age at the onset of signs and symptoms in children is 9.5 years. Tumors arising in the adrenal medulla produce both epinephrine and norepinephrine, whereas most extra-adrenal pheochromocytomas produce only norepinephrine. The catecholamines released by the tumors may directly or indirectly activate that alpha- and/or beta-adrenergic receptors, resulting in apprehension, hypertension, tachycardia, diaphoresis, evidence of increased metabolism, constipation, gastrointestinal bleeding, and other symptoms. A functioning pheochromocytoma usually causes sustained hypertension in children, in contrast to adults, who generally have paroxysmal elevations of blood pressure. Episodes of tachycardia, systolic hypertension, and arrhythmias reflect the muscular beta-receptor effects of epinephrine secretion, whereas bradycardia and diastolic hypertension are evidence of increased peripheral vasoconstriction by alpha-receptors from circulating norepinephrine. A contracted vascular system often results, owing to decreased plasma volume, reduced red cell mass, and occasionally, orthostatic hypotension [10]. Norepinephrine is predominantly alpha in effect, whereas epinephrine elicits a mixture of alpha and beta actions. The majority of childhood pheochromocytomas contain, but do not secrete, substantial quantities of dopamine, which is primarily a beta-stimulator. The relative proportions of norepinephrine and epinephrine may influence the signs and symptoms produced by pheochromocytomas [11]. In general, higher levels of norepinephrine are encountered in most childhood tumors, possibly reflecting a higher incidence of extra-adrenal pheochromocytomas, which do not possess the capacity for methylation of norepinephrine.

The onset of symptoms in children is often rapid, with diaphoresis unrelated to environmental temperature, usually preceded by pallor. Throbbing headaches with flushing may occur, and hands may show a puffy redness, cyanosis, and mottling. Elevated body temperature, dilated pupils, and heat intolerance may become evident. Weight loss is common, despite a ravenous appetite. Occasionally, substernal, precordial, abdominal, lumbar, or femoral pain may be present as a constant or colicky symptom. Epistaxis, hematemesis, melena, nausea and vomiting may be associated with abdominal pain, which may simulate or actually be caused by colitis or appendicitis [12]. Partial intestinal obstruction may stem from fecal impaction. Polyuria, polydipsia, microscopic hematuria, and glycosuria with elevated fasting blood sugar levels are typical of pheochromocytoma in children and adults. Convulsions and coma may occasionally result from hypertensive encephalopathy, and vision may be blurred by hypertensive retinitis. Despite these alarming symptoms, sudden death due to pheochromocytoma is uncommon in childhood. Peripheral vasoconstriction, bradycardia, and sweating characterize the alpha effects, while the beta effects include tachycardia, increased cardiac contractile force, bronchodilatation, and peripheral vasodilatation with lowered diastolic blood pressure.

Hypertension from pheochromocytomas may be differentiated from that due to coarctation of the aorta by the presence of bounding femoral pulses in pheochromocytoma. Many renal lesions, including intrinsic and extrinsic tumors, unilateral and bilateral pyelonephritis, glomerulonephritis, and renal artery stenosis may be associated with hypertension in childhood. Urinalysis, renal function studies, MRI scan, and arteriography can, in most cases, distinguish these conditions from pheochromocytoma. Other causes of hypertension in childhood that should be differentiated from pheochromocytoma are hyperthyroidism, adrenogenital syndrome, Cushing's syndrome, acrodynia, brain tumor, lead poisoning and essential hypertension. In children with paroxysmal hypertension, the diagnosis of familial autonomic dysfunction (Riley-Day syndrome) should be ruled out.

Approximately 10% of childhood pheochromocytomas are familial, four times the frequency in adults. This familial occurrence has been noted in a variety of syndromes that are attributed to genetic derangements of neural crest derivatives. The common cell origin of a number of endocrine tumors was regarded by Pearse as a part of the neuroendocrine group; on the basis of the function of the cells, he termed these "APUD tumors" (amine precursor uptake and decarboxylation) [13]. These cells are believed to be totipotential, migratory, and capable of secreting a variety of polypeptide hormones [14].

Sipple's syndrome, multiple endocrine adenomatosis II (MEA II), and multiple endocrine neoplasia (MEN II) are genetic disorders involving multifocal tumor formation in the system of polypeptide-secreting cells. Their expressions can include pheochromocytoma, medullary carcinoma of the thyroid, parathyroid hyperplasia or tumors, and multiple mucosal neuromas [14]. The neuroma associated with Sipple's syndrome develops primarily in the lip and is a true neuroma rather than the nerve sheath tumor that characterizes Recklinghausen's disease. Patients whose disease complex is characterized by medullary carcinoma of the thyroid, by pheochromocytoma, by multiple mucosal neuroma of the lips, tongue and upper eyelids, and by pathognomonic facies are subclassified as MEA IIb [15]. These patients also commonly have a marfanoid habitus. The only true clinical overlap with Recklinghausen's neurofibromatosis is the association of pheochromocytoma, usually bilateral.

Adrenal medullary hyperplasia has been documented as a probable precursor of pheochromocytoma in the MEA II syndrome [16]. Serum calcitonin determinations have been used for screening potential MEA II patients for medullary thyroid cancers. In occult cases, the pentagastrin-stimulation test of calcitonin secretion may prove more reliable [11]. The association of pheochromocytoma with parathyroid hyperplasia or adenomas in the MEA II syndrome may be secondary or compensatory in nature, representing reactive stimulation of the parathyroid to maintain normal calcium concentrations in response to the calcium-lowering effects of calcitonin.

Approximately 4% of patients with pheochromocytomas have accompanying neurocutaneous syndromes, including Recklinghausen's disease, tuberous sclerosis, Sturge-Weber syndrome, and von Hippel-Lindau disease [15]. The 12% incidence of other anomalies in such children's families (hydrocephalus, neurofibromas, ganglioneuromas, megacolon megaureter, cryptorchidism) suggests a genetic trait having characteristics of a malformation syndrome. The incidence of pheochromocytoma is increased in patients suffering from congenital heart disease.

Diagnostic studies

Since many pheochromocytomas in children are extra-adrenal or bilateral, preoperative localization of the tumor is critical to safe, expeditious surgical management. Abdominal ultrasonography, computed tomography (CT), and/or magnetic resonance imaging (MRI) can contribute to localizing a pheochromocytoma. Intravenous pyelography may be helpful in the case of large adrenal tumors. Aortography with selective arterial catheterization may be helpful in the rare child whose tumor is not discoverable through less invasive studies, although this procedure serves as a provocative test which may produce paroxysmal catecholamine release, and precautions must therefore be taken to manage reactions (Fig. 1). The presence of functional chromaffin tissue can be detected by iodine-131 iobenguane (^{131}I-metaiodobenzylguanidine) [17]. This guanidine analogue has a molecular structure similar to that of norepinephrine and is concentrated in catecholamine storage vesicles. It has been particularly useful in localizing extra-adrenal and recurrent pheochromocytomas. Any child suspected of having a pheochromocytoma should be evaluated in a hospital setting where accurate urine collection is feasible and the hazards of special procedures can be minimized. Overzealous and prolonged diagnostic efforts to localize a tumor may seriously delay treatment.

The histamine provocative test and other tests to increase catecholamine secretion have been eliminated from the diagnostic armamentarium because of risks associated with increasing catecholamine secretion in an already hyper-

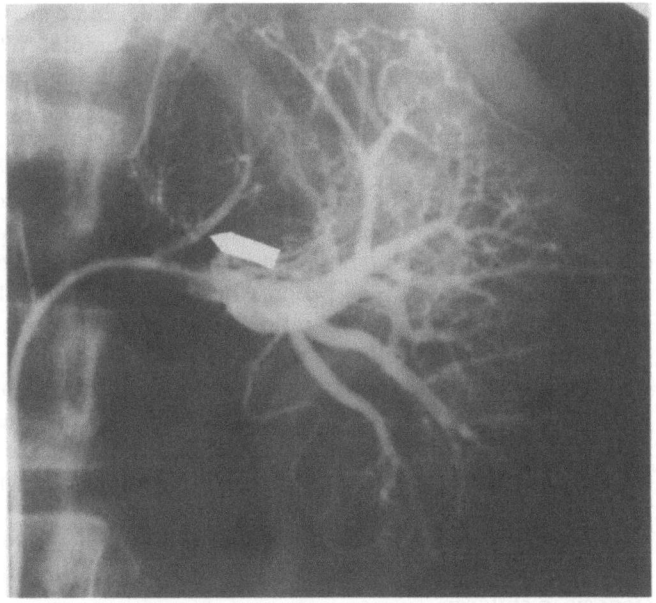

Fig. 1. Left renal arteriogram showing arterial circulation to large left adrenal pheochromocytoma

tensive patient. The phentolamine (Regitine) test is useful only in patients with sustained hypertension and should rarely be used. A positive result produces a 25–35 mm Hg fall of pressure within 5–10 min after intravenous injection of 5 mg Regitine.

During the past few years, direct chemical methods of measuring catecholamine levels and metabolites in plasma have largely replaced the indirect pharmacologic tests. Catecholamine secretion is initiated by acetylcholine released from neurons that embrace the secretory cell. After a brief period of activity in the circulation, these catecholamines are reduced by oxidation to 3-methoxy, 4-hydroxy-mandelic acid (VMA). Only 2%–4% of norepinephrine and epinephrine is excreted directly into the urine, whereas more than one third of the total secreted catecholamine appears as VMA and one half is excreted as free or conjugated metanephrines [18]. A direct linear relation between the rate of urinary excretion of VMA and the size of a pheochromocytoma has been reported [19]. Because of their higher concentrations, urinary assays for the metabolites of the epinephrine or norepinephrine has proved easier and more reliable. A pheochromocytoma may be localized by determining catecholamine levels in blood samples obtained at various levels in the inferior vena cava when not identified by MRI studies.

The most commonly used diagnostic tests in children are 24-h collections of urine for free catecholamines, VMA, and metanephrines. For screening purposes, overnight urine collection can be used. The catecholamine quantities are modified by the amount of creatinine in the sample. When the total catechol- amine level is normal, epinephrine-norepinephrine fractionation has proved highly reliable [20]. An increased epinephrine fraction (> 20%) may help in iden- tifying a pheochromocytoma. Although VMA assays are widely available, they are subject to interference from various medications and dietary components. Assays of urinary catecholamines and VMA have been associated with an approx- imate 25% incidence of false-negative findings, whereas such results occurred in only 4% of metanephrine determinations. Measurement of urinary homovanillic acid (HVA), the major end product of dopamine metabolism, may help to diag- nose malignant dopamine-secreting pheochromocytomas. Patients with neuro- blastoma characteristically secrete high levels of dopamine metabolites.

Measurement of plasma catecholamines by radioisotope enzyme assay may be more effective than either 24-h urinary VMA or metanephrine determinations [21]. Patients must remain supine while blood samples are obtained; nonetheless, the catecholamine assay offers the major advantage of obviating 24-h urine collec- tion, which can be difficult in young children.

Plasma renin activity may increase in approximately 70% of patients with pheochromocytomas, possibly leading to an erroneous diagnosis of renal artery stenosis in children.

Treatment

Medical therapy for children with functioning pheochromocytomas is limited al- most exclusively to preoperative preparation. Phentolamine and phenoxybenz- amine (Dibenzyline) act to block the alpha-adrenergic receptors of epinephrine and norepinephrine. Because of the potential danger of hypertensive paroxysms, the patient should be started on alpha-blocking agents as soon as the diagnosis of pheochromocytoma has been confirmed. Phenoxybenzamine is the most effective alpha-adrenergic blocker, because its 12- to 24-h duration of action allows oral administration twice daily. The recommended starting dose of phenoxybenzamine is 1–2 mg/kg/24 h in four divided doses; the dose should be increased until the blood pressure returns to normal. Phentolamine can be used for rapid alpha- adrenergic blockade, whereas phenoxybenzamine therapy for 1–2 weeks can be employed when surgery is not urgent. Congestion of nasal mucosa is a minor side effect. Prazosin is a new drug under trial which specifically blocks only the post- synaptic alpha-1 receptors and has fewer side effects than phenoxybenzamine [20].

The beta-adrenergic blocker, propranolol, has been used to prepare patients for operation, or intraoperatively to control tachycardia and prevent arrhythmias resulting from alpha-adrenergic blockade. Routine preoperative use of beta blockade has been somewhat controversial since occasional severe cardiovascular crises have occurred after its use. Nitroprusside has occasionally been used both preoperatively and intraoperatively in patients who have become refractory to oral and intravenous alpha blockers. Patients with pheochromocytomas tend to be hypovolemic, experiencing an average 15% reduction of normal plasma volume. Carefully monitored preoperative re-expansion of the vascular system helps to minimize intraoperative fluctuations in blood pressure and intractable cardiac arrhythmias. Use of drugs that decrease catecholamine synthesis, such as alpha-methylparathyrosine (AMPT), an inhibitor of tyrosine hydroxylase, has been recommended as an alternative preoperative treatment regimen [17]. Prolonged medical therapy has no place in the current treatment of pheochromocytomas.

Children with pheochromocytoma who have a high basal metabolic rate and high plasma level of catecholamines have generally been recognized as the poorest anesthesia risks. General anesthesia for excision of a pheochromocytoma may be divided into two stages. The first is characterized by efforts to keep the systemic blood pressure down while the tumor is isolated and its blood supply is ligated. The second involves efforts to keep the systemic blood pressure up thereafter. For safe anesthetic management, it is essential to use arterial and central venous pressure catheters as well as a urinary catheter, and to monitor the electrocardiogram continuously. The following drugs should be available to reduce systemic hypertension: phentolamine, nitroprusside, and diazoxide. To control tachycardia and cardia arrhythmias, Xylocaine and propranolol are necessary. It is recommended that the anesthesiologist accompany the patient from the ward and administer 0.04 ml/kg Innovar intravenously at that time, repeating the dose after 5 min if the patient remains anxious.

The induction of general anesthesia is particularly critical, because inadequate sedation may produce severe hypertension, while excessive alpha blockade with inadequate blood volume re-expansion may result in severe hypotension. Enflurane has become the anesthetic drug of choice in recent years, although the plane of anesthesia is probably more important than the agent employed. Enflurane does not sensitize the myocardium to exogenous catecholamines, nor does it stimulate the release of catecholamines. Pancuronium, a nondepolarizing, long-acting muscle relaxant administered intravenously, is preferred over succinylcholine or curare. After intubation, anesthesia can also be maintained by a combination of nitrous oxide and oxygen with methoxyflurane. Innovar may also be administered if additional analgesia is required during operation. Halothane is not employed because of its propensity to sensitize the myocardium to the arrhythmic activity of catecholamines. Blood and, if necessary, norepinephrine or angiotensin II should be used to control hypotension that may occur precipitously after removal of the tumor [14].

Since more than 95% of childhood pheochromocytomas are located in the abdomen, although the tumor site may occasionally be inaccurately determined, a bilateral subcostal incision that can be extended into the flank or into the chest for large tumors has provided satisfactory exposure. Abdominal exploration including direct visualization of both adrenal glands, the periaortic sympathetic ganglia, the small-bowel mesentery, and the pelvis will reveal almost all pheochromocytomas in children. Gentle dissection with early control of venous drainage and minimal manipulation of the tumor or involved gland should be employed to avoid flooding the circulation with excess catecholamines. The tumor is usually encapsulated and may have small remnants of normal adrenal tissue contiguous with it. The entire adrenal gland should be removed. Pheochromocytomas rarely adhere to the kidney, so that a concomitant nephrectomy is seldom required. Clear visualization and exploration of the contralateral adrenal gland is mandatory for all children because of the high incidence of bilateral tumors. When the adrenal veins are divided and the pheochromocytoma is removed, hypotension usually ensues, requiring a norepinephrine infusion for varying periods of time, ranging up to several days. The reduced blood volume resulting from long-term catecholamine secretion should be corrected by appropriate transfusions of plasma, albumin, blood, or electrolyte solutions, as indicated. Adrenocortical insufficiency is unlikely if the major portion of one adrenal gland is left in place. If both adrenals are removed, or if the remaining gland is atrophic, intravenous hydrocortisone should be given promptly.

In the occasional child the blood pressure may not return to a normal level for several days after tumor removal. In our clinical experience with resection of pheochromocytomas in 17 children, when blood pressure failed to normalize within 2–3 weeks, or when hypertension returned, a second tumor was often found. Hypertension due to a second pheochromocytoma is apt to occur within 5 years subsequent to removal of the initial tumor. Children who undergo resection of the pheochromocytoma should have follow-up examinations at least twice annually, including measurement of blood pressure and urine catecholamine determinations. The progeny and siblings of patients with pheochromocytoma should also be periodically evaluated for hypertension because of the high familial incidence.

Although malignancy of pheochromocytomas is approximately 10% in adults, it is uncommon in children and is usually diagnosed by the finding of distant nonfunctioning metastases. On the basis of its histology, it is difficult to predict whether a pheochromocytoma in a child will behave as a malignant tumor, since pleomorphism and lymphatic, vascular, and capsular invasion are frequently evident. A combination of local excision, radiation, chemotherapy, and antiadrenergic agents has provided symptomatic palliation for many years in these rare patients. Complete cure is difficult to achieve.

References

1. Frankel F (1986) Ein Fall von doppelseitigen, völlig latent verlaufenen Nebennierentumor und gleichzeitiger Nephritis mit Veränderungen am Circulationsapparat und Retinitis. Arch Pathol Anat 103:244–249
2. Labbe M, Tinel J, Doumer A (1922) Crises solaires et hypertension paroxysmique en rapport avec une tumeur surrenale. Bull Soc Med Hop Paris 46:982–987
3. Pick L (1912) Das Ganglioma Embryonale Sympathicum. Klin Wochenschr 19:16–22
4. Kremer DN (1936) Medullary tumor of the adrenal glands. Arch Intern Med 57:999–1005
5. Stackpole RH, Melicow MM, Uson SC (1963) Pheochromocytoma in children: report of nine cases with follow-up studies. J Pediatr Surg 63:314–319
6. Kvale WF, Roth GM, Manager WM, et al (1957) Present-day diagnosis and treatment of pheochromocytoma. JAMA 164:854–860

7. Hume DM (1960) Pheochromocytoma in the adult and in the child. Am J Surg 99:458–466
8. Bloom DA, Fonkalsrud EW (1974) Surgical management of pheochromocytoma in children. J Pediatr Surg 9:179–184
9. Gibbs MK, Carney JA, Hayles AB, et al (1977) Simultaneous adrenal and cerivcal pheochromocytomas in childhood. Ann Surg 185:273–278
10. Brunjes J, Johns VJ Jr, Crane MD (1960) Pheochromocytoma: postoperative shock and blood volume. N Engl J Med 262:393–397
11. Dibbins AW, Wiener ES (1973) Retroperitoneal tumors in children. Curr Probl Surg 10 (10):318–346
12. Fee HJ, Fonkalsrud EW, Ament ME, et al (1975) Enterocolitis with peritonitis in a child with pheochromocytoma. Ann Surg 185:448–450
13. Scott HW Jr, Oates JA, Nies AS, et al (1976) Pheochromocytoma: present diagnosis and management. Ann Surg 183:587–593
14. Stringel G, Ein SH, Creighton R, et al (1980) Pheochromocytoma in children: an update. J Pediatr Surg 15:496–500
15. Van Heerden JA, Shops SG, Hamberger B, et al (1982) Pheochromocytoma: current status and changing trends. Surgery 91:367–372
16. Carney JA, Sizemore GW, Tyce GM (1975) Bilateral adrenal medullary hyperplasia in multiple endocrine neoplasia, type II: The precursor of bilateral pheochromocytoma. Mayo Clin Proc 50:3–8
17. Sisson JL, Frager MS, Valk TW, et al (1981) Scintigraphic localization of pheochromocytoma. N Engl J Med 305:12–17
18. Javadpour N, Woltering EA, Brennan MF (1980) Adrenal neoplasm. Curr Probl Surg 17:349–385
19. Farndon JR, Davidson HA, Johnson IDA, et al (1980) VMA excretion in patients with pheochromocytoma. Ann Surg 191:259–264
20. Havlik RJ, Cahow CE, Kinder BK (1988) Advances in the diagnosis and treatment of pheochromocytoma. Arch Surg 123:626–630
21. Bravo EL, Tarazi RC, Gifford RW, et al (1979) Circulating and urinary catecholamines in pheochromocytoma. N Engl J Med 301:682–687

Surgical Treatment of Ovarian Tumors in Childhood

M. G. Schwöbel and U. G. Stauffer

Summary

From 1971 to 1988, 45 girls aged 1 week to 17 years were treated for a total of 46 solid and cystic tumors of the ovaries. Pathohistological examination revealed epithelial tumors in eight cases, a tumor originating from the ovarian stroma in one case, germinal tumors in 17 cases, 15 functional ovarian cysts, and five paraovarian cysts. The stroma tumor and four of the 17 germinal tumors were malignant. Surgical treatment for solid tumors consisted generally of a unilateral salpingo-oophorectomy, but in operations for cystic tumors as well, vital ovarian tissue could only rarely be preserved. Functional ovarian cysts were excised if they were larger than 5 cm. Subsequent to excision of malignant tumors, chemotherapy with cisplatin, vincristine and bleomycin was performed. On follow-up, all patients with benign lesions were well. One of the girls with malignancies died and another is undergoing chemotherapy for tumor recurrence in the contralateral ovary.

Zusammenfassung

Von 1971 bis 1988 wurden 45 Mädchen im Alter von 1 Woche bis 17 Jahren wegen 46 solider oder zystischer Ovarialtumoren behandelt. Es handelte sich um 8 epitheliale Tumoren, einen vom gonadalen Stroma ausgehenden Tumor, 17 Keimzelltumoren, 15 funktionelle Ovarialzysten und 5 Paraovarialzysten. Der Stromatumor und 4 der Keimzelltumoren waren maligne.

Die chirurgische Therapie der soliden Tumoren bestand in der Regel aus der unilateralen Salpingo-Oophorektomie. Aber auch bei der Operation zystischer Tumoren konnte nur selten vitales Ovargewebe erhalten werden. Funktionelle Ovarialzysten wurden operiert, wenn sie größer als 5 cm waren.

Nach der Resektion maligner Tumoren wurde eine Chemotherapie mit Cisplatin, Vincristin und Bleomycin angeschlossen. Die Patientinnen mit benignen Läsionen sind bei der Nachkontrolle alle beschwerdefrei. Von den Mädchen mit malignen Tumoren ist eines gestorben und ein zweites steht wegen eines Rezidivs im Gegenovar unter Chemotherapie.

Résumé

Entre 1971 et 1988 nous avons traité 45 fillettes âgées de 1 semaine à 17 ans pour 46 tumeurs ovariennes solides ou kystiques. Il s'agissait de 8 tumeurs épithéliales, d'une tumeur provenant d'un stroma gonadique, de 17 tumeurs des cellules germinatives, de 15 kystes ovariens fonctionnels et de 5 kystes paroovariens. La tumeur du stroma et 4 des tumeurs des cellules germinatives étaient malignes.

Le traitement chirurgical des tumeurs solides consistait en règle générale en une salpingo-ovarectomie (oophorectomie). Lors de la résection de tumeurs kystiques, il n'était que rarement

Pediatric Surgical Clinic, University Children's Hospital of Zurich, Steinwiesstraße 75, CH-8032 Zurich, Switzerland.

Progress in Pediatric Surgery, Vol. 26
Gauderer and Angerpointner (Eds.)
© Springer-Verlag Berlin Heidelberg 1991

possible de conserver du tissu ovarien vital. Les kystes ovarien ont été opérés quand leur taille dépassait 5 cm.

Après la résection des tumeurs malignes, il y eut une chimiothérapie au cis-platinum, à la vincristine et à la bléomycine. Les patients n'ayant que des lésions bénignes ne présentaient plus aucun symptôme au contôle ultérieur. Une des fillettes ayant une tumeur maligne est décédée et une autre subit une chimiothérapie pour une récidive dans l'autre ovaire.

Introduction

Ovarian surgery in childhood is only seldom necessary [16]. Nevertheless, knowledge of the pathology and pathophysiology of the female gonad is important for the pediatric surgeon to make the correct diagnostic and therapeutic decisions when confronted with pathological conditions of the ovaries.

We present our therapeutic procedure and its results in girls with tumors or tumor-like lesions of the ovaries. Patients who underwent diagnostic laparotomies for polycystic ovaries or endocrine problems are excluded. We use the WHO classification, shown in Table 1.

Patients

A total of 46 ovarian tumors or cysts were operated in 45 patients between January 1971 and December 1988. One girl had to operated on twice within 2 years for two different findings.

The average of one to two patients per year remained constant for many years, but recently ovarian surgery in children has increased significantly (Fig. 1). This is due to the routine use of ultrasound as a screening method for abdominal complaints of unclear origin. Surprisingly, however, the number of patients with malignant ovarian tumors has also increased.

The age at operation is shown in Fig. 2. Remarkably, prenatal diagnosis of a pathological finding of the ovary was made in one case only, and surgery was per-

Table 1. Pathohistological classification of ovarian tumors (WHO 1973)

I	Common epithelial tumors, e.g., serous cystadenoma
II	Tumors of the ovarian stroma, e.g., granulosa cell tumor
III	Lipoid cell tumors
IV	Germinal tumors, e.g., dysgerminoma, mature and immature teratoma, endodermal sinus tumor
V	Mixed germinal and ovarian stroma tumors, e.g., gonadoblastoma
VI	Soft-tissue tumors not specific for the ovary, such as fibroma, myxoma
VII	Unclassified tumors
VIII	Secondary tumors (metastases), e.g., malignant lymphoma [14]
IX	Tumor-like lesions, e.g., follicular cyst, corpus luteum cyst, paraovarian cyst

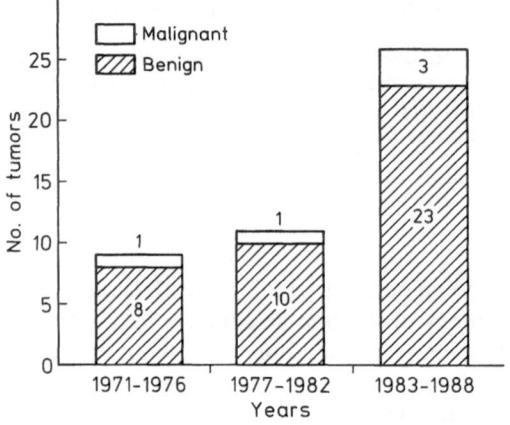

Fig. 1. Increase in ovarian tumors and cysts among children over three consecutive 5-year periods

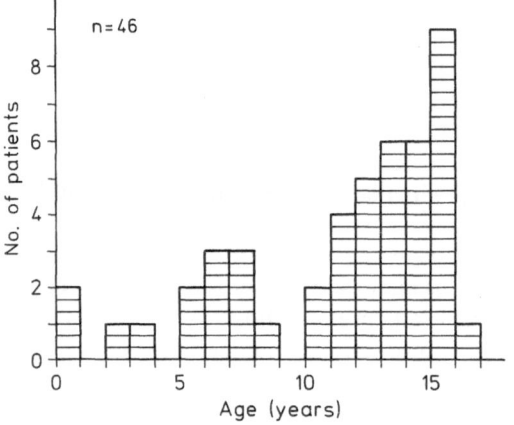

Fig. 2. Age at operation of 46 patients with ovarian tumors 1971–1988

formed during the first year of life in only two cases. There is a minor peak between the 6th and 8th year of life, due to a prevalence of benign ovarian teratomas in this age group. The number of patients rises steeply after menarche because of an increase of ovarian cysts.

Eighteen girls suffered from solid or mainly solid ovarian tumors, five of which were malignant. Nearly two thirds of the pathological entities were cystic lesions. The pathohistological findings in our cases are summarized in Table 2.

Acute abdominal pain was the leading symptom in more than half of the girls with ovarian and paraovarian cysts. A palpable mass, on the other hand, predominated in girls with ovarian teratomas and cystadenomas [1]. Premature thelarche combined with vaginal discharge occurred in only two girls with ovarian cysts. These two ovarian cysts, one malignant ovarian teratoma, and two yolk sac tumors were endocrine active.

Table 2. Histological diagnosis of 46 pathological ovarian lesions in 45 girls

Serous cystadenoma and cystadenofibroma (benign)	8
Malignant neuroectodermal tumor	1
Benign teratoma (dermoid cyst)	13
Malignant teratoma	2
Endodermal sinus tumor (yolk sac tumor)	2
Functional ovarian cysts	15
Paraovarian cysts	5
Total	46

Epithelial Tumors

The only epithelial tumors occurring in our patients were cystadenomas and cystadenofibromas. Eight girls between 5 and 16 years were thus affected. Remarkably, the tumor site was the right ovary in seven cases. In all but one case, the cystic part predominated, containing up to 2.5 l fluid. Numerous small cysts and interstitial fibrosis were found in the remaining case, pathohistologically corresponding to a cystadenofibroma. In two cases the cysts could be enucleated from the remaining ovary, and the organ was thus preserved. In the other cases ovarian tissue had entirely disappeared because of the pressure exerted by the cyst. This was confirmed histologically.

Although the adenocarcinoma is the most common ovarian tumor in mature women, particularly after menopause, carcinomas of the ovaries practically never occur in childhood and there were none in our patients. Likewise, no ovarian carcinomas in women under 20 years of age were reported to the registry of the workshop of the Swiss Gynecological Hospitals (1983–1986) [3]. Cronen and Nagaraj [7] described only one girl with a cystadenocarcinoma among 30 patients with ovarian tumors. Ehren et al. [6] found only one cystadenocarcinoma in 63 children with ovarian tumors; this girl already had liver metastases and died 12 days following surgery.

Tumors of the Ovarian Stroma

The granulosa cell tumors and Sertoli-Leydig cell tumors belong to this group. Combinations with germinal tumors and undifferentiated tumors are very rare [19]. Granulosa cell tumors appear typically in young adults, and we have not seen a case with this tumor type at our hospital during the past 18 years. These tumors are frequently endocrine active and exhibit a relatively benign course. Therefore, unilateral salpingo-oophorectomy is generally sufficient [2]. Vassal et al. [34] reported on 15 girls with granulosa cell tumors whom they had treated over a period of 19 years. Eleven of the patients are free of recurrence an average of 6 years following surgery. In four cases where the tumors had primarily invaded the surrounding structures the patients developed recurrences, and all have died.

We have recently seen a case of a bilateral, malignant, undifferenciated stroma cell tumor. The medical course will be briefly described. The 12.5-year-old girl was repeatedly seen at our outpatient department for familial gigantism during the year prior to her hospitalization. The last examination, 3 months prior to the acute onset of illness, had not revealed any pathological findings. Endocrinological examinations had not been performed. The onset of menarche was at the age of 11 years, 10 months. During summer vacation in Italy the girl had to be hospitalized for acute dyspnea. Clinical examinations revealed bilateral pneumonia, bilateral pleural effusions, and ascites. After 1 week without clinical improvement she was flown back to Switzerland. Shortly after admission to our hospital she had to be intubated and artificially ventilated. Further diagnosis disclosed bilateral ovarian tumors with metastases in the retroperitoneum, lungs, pleura, base and vault of the skull, and bone marrow. The alpha-fetoprotein (AFP) was normal, but beta-human-chorionic gonadotropin (HCG), at 31 IU/l, was slightly increased (normal range, 0–5 IU/l). A bilateral ovariectomy was carried out. The right ovary weighed 470 g, the left 300 g. Chemotherapy with actinomycin D, cyclophosphamide and vincristine was started subsequent to surgery. There was no response, and the girl died on the tenth postoperative day of multiorgan failure. Pathohistological examination revealed a parvicellular stroma cell tumor. Electron-microscopical and immunohistochemical examinations showed a neuroectodermal tumor.

Germinal Tumors

Teratomas

Fifteen girls aged 2–16 years were operated on for ovarian teratomas. The weight of the tumors ranged from 60 to 2800 g; there was no prevalence of the left or right side. Treatment consisted of a unilateral ovariectomy in 14 patients and enucleation of a predominantly cystic teratoma with preservation of the ovary in the remaining patient. Two teratomas were malignant. The medical histories of these two patients are described here in brief.

T. M., 12 years, 3 months. The patient became aware of an increase in her abdominal circumference 4 weeks prior to hospitalization. Except for a feeling of pressure, she had no other symptoms. Clinical examination revealed a huge palpable mass extending from the xiphoid process to the symphysis and into both flanks. A tumor weighing 2800 g and originating from the right ovary was removed in toto by laparotomy via a lower transverse approach. Histologically, the tumor was found to be a malignant teratoma, limited to the organ itself. There was no evidence of local or remote metastases. The girl is doing well 7 years following the operation and subsequent chemotherapy with vincristine, actinomycin D, and cyclophosphamide.

B. C., 6 years, 1 month. The girl underwent laparotomy at a district hospital at the age of 6 years and 1 month for acute abdominal pain and suspected acute appendicitis. A tumor originating from the right ovary was found and subtotally removed. Peritoneal metastases were already present. Subsequent to surgery, irradiation therapy with a total dose of 3000 rads was carried out. However, the girl developed a recurrent tumor 5 months following surgery and was transferred to our hospital. The AFP was normal, but the beta-HCG, at 10600 IU/l, was markedly elevated prior to surgery. On laparotomy, the recurrent tumor weighing 750 g was removed. Radical tumor excision was again impossible. Further tumor growth could be prevented by means of chemotherapy with cyclophosphamide and vincristine combined with intra-abdominal implantation of radiogold. The woman is free of recurrence today, 18 years after the first operation, and can be regarded as cured. Remarkably, menarche took place and further development was entirely normal. She is taking contraceptives, as a child is not desired so far.

Larger series also report malignancy in $\frac{1}{5}$ to $\frac{1}{6}$ of all teratomas [5, 15, 20, 32]. Billmire and Grosfeld [4] reported on ovarian teratomas in 15 patients they had seen between 1960 and 1984, of which 11 were benign and four malignant. Only one of the malignant tumors could be excised in toto; the patient was symptom free at follow-up. The remaining malignant teratomas not radically removable metastasized rapidly, and all patients died.

Dysgerminoma

According to La Vecchia et al. [20] and Breen and Maxson [5], dysgerminomas are five times as frequent as teratomas. Nevertheless, we saw no patient with a dysgerminoma between 1971 and 1988. Steck [31] summarized all patients with ovarian tumors treated at our hospital from 1934 to 1954. Among those 19 patients, one girl had a dysgerminoma. This tumor is histologically identical and embryologically equivalent to the testicular seminoma. Five to twenty percent of dysgerminomas occur bilaterally [5]. Since the prognosis depends largely on tumor stage at the primary operation, standardized surgical procedures and peritoneal lavage for intraoperative cytological sampling are necessary [33]. Weinblatt and Ortega [35] recommend a unilateral salpingo-oophorectomy for a stage-IA tumor according to FIGO [12] and a bilateral salpingo-oophorectomy with hysterectomy for stage IB. Only if the tumor extends beyond the organ borders is chemotherapy given subsequent to surgery. Although the dysgerminoma is the only ovarian tumor really sensitive to radiotherapy, irradiation was applied as the primary treatment in only two of nine patients by these authors. If the tumor does not extend beyond the organ borders, cure can be expected in over 90% of cases [10].

Endodermal Sinus (Yolk Sac) Tumor

In large series the endodermal sinus tumor appears as the third most common ovarian tumor [5, 20]. The age peak is at around 20 years, but it has also been observed in young children. Rapid invasion of the pelvic organs and early metastasis render this tumor highly malignant. In the series of Kurman and Norris [18], only 13% of the patients survived longer than 3 years. We saw two girls with endodermal sinus tumors during the period under discussion.

S. S., 7 years, 2 months. The girl had suffered from diffuse abdominal pain and dysuria for 1 week before hospitalization. Urinalysis was normal. Symptomatic therapy did not improve the girl's condition. She was admitted to the hospital because of a palpable mass the size of a child's head in the lower abdomen. Ultrasound and CT increased the suspicion of a malignant tumor originating from the ovaries or the uterus, but the primarily affected organ could not be exactly specified. On laparotomy a 350-g tumor was found, originating from the left ovary and adhering to the bladder wall. It was excised in toto, together with the bladder wall. Pathohistological examination revealed an endodermal sinus tumor. The bladder wall was tumor free, and the tumor was classified as stage I. Postoperative chemotherapy with vincristine, actinomycin D, and cyclophosphamide was carried out. An increase of serum AFP to 1968 IU/ml (normal range up to 20 IU/ml) was diagnosed 9 months after salpingo-oophorectomy. Radiology disclosed a tumor recurrence in the uterus and right ovary. Relaparotomy disclosed peritoneal carcinosis as well, and a right-sided salpingo-oophorectomy and hysterectomy was performed. Postoperative chemotherapy consisted of cisplatin, bleomycin, and vinblastine. AFP dropped to normal postoperatively and remains normal 4 months following surgery.

M. M., 15 years, 6 months. The girl complained of diffuse abdominal pain and a feeling of pressure 1 month prior to hospitalization. When she could no longer close her trousers, she went to see a physician, who diagnosed ascites and sent her to the hospital. Clinical and radiological examinations revealed ascites, a right-sided pleural effusion, and a vaginally and rectally clearly palpable tumor in the lower abdomen. At 3353 IU/ml (normal up to 20 IU/ml) serum AFP was markedly elevated, the beta-HCG at 6 IU/l (normal up to 5 IU/l) slightly elevated. On laparotomy, 5 l of ascitic fluid was aspirated and the tumor, originating from the right ovary, was removed. The left ovary was macroscopically and histologically tumor free. Likewise, no malignant cells were found in the ascitic fluid. The girl recovered quickly and the ascites and pleural effusion did not reappear. Serum AFP and beta-HCG levels were normal 1 month following surgery. Today, 4 months after the operation, the girl is undergoing chemotherapy with carboplatin, vinblastine, and bleomycin. She is radiologically and clinically without evidence of a recurrence.

Tumor-like Lesions

Functional Cysts

Follicular and corpus luteum cysts are regarded as functional cysts. Whereas corpus luteum cysts occur only in sexually mature girls, follicular cysts are seen in any age-group. We subdivided our patients into three age-groups, namely neonatal, childhood up to puberty, and post-menarche.

Neonatal

Two infant girls belonged to this group. R. C. was delivered via cesarean section in the 27th gestational week because of pre-term labor and was immediately intubated for 27 hours thereafter. Prematurity problems were overcome during the next several weeks. Apneic spells were treated with theophylline. At the age of 4 months, 2 weeks after term, an endocrinological examination was performed for grossly feminized external genitalia and vaginal discharge. The estrogens were markedly elevated (E2 380 pg/ml; E3 180 pg/ml). Abdominal ultrasound disclosed a large cyst in the right adnexa. On subsequent laparotomy, the cyst, which had destroyed the ovarian tissue, was removed and small cysts were enucleated from the left ovary. Pathohistological examination disclosed follicular cysts on the right as well as on the left side. The external genitalia normalized entirely postoperatively. However, the E2 and E3 remained slightly elevated even 6 months after operation.

Antenatal ultrasound performed in the 39th gestational week revealed an intra-abdominal cyst 8×9 cm in the girl R. M., 1 week prior to delivery. Postnatally, there was a fist-sized palpable mass in the right lower and middle abdomen of the otherwise healthy baby. At laparotomy performed on the 4th day of life, a 360° twisted ovarian cyst was found. The right fallopian tube was infarcted and histological examination revealed no vital ovarian tissue.

Gaudin et al. [11] reported on 11 children with antenatally diagnosed ovarian cysts. Six girls with minor cysts were observed with ultrasound monitoring, and the cysts disappeared during the first year of life. Five girls with cysts measuring 3.5–6 cm in diameter were operated on. The authors found antenatally contorted cysts that had destroyed the ovarian tissue in all cases.

Frémond et al. [9] described ten children, nine of whom had cysts between 40 and 90 mm in diameter and were operated on. Five of these cysts were twisted and had effected necrosis of the ovary. Only one child was observed over time, and the 35-mm cyst disappeared spontaneously. Zachariou et al. [36] operated on seven girls shortly after birth in whom ovarian cysts had been diagnosed antenatally. Salpingo-oophorectomy was carried out in all cases, and vital ovarian tissue was found in none. One girl developed an additional complication, insofar as the cyst had led to small bowel necrosis. Scholz et al. [28] reported on a similar complication. In their patient a large ovarian cyst had caused a perforation of the cecum. All these cysts were observed in term babies and were endocrine inactive. Sedin et al. [29] published reports of four girls delivered before the 30th gestational week in whom estradiol-producing ovarian cysts were found 1–4 weeks before term. One of these cysts was surgically removed, two disappeared spontaneously, and two were treated with medroxyprogesterone acetate (one was on the contralateral ovary of the girl who was operated on). Measurements of serum LH and FSH levels after LHRH stimulation showed autonomous estradiol production by the cysts. Our patient R. C., who was also born prior to the 30th gestational week, likewise exhibited autonomous estradiol production by the ovarian cysts. Moreover, the patients of Sedin et al. and our patient have in common that all received theophylline for apneic spells. However, nothing is found in the literature with regard to induction of ovarian cysts by theophylline. Hormone-producing ovarian cysts appear predominantly in term girls with diabetic mothers [13].

There is no general agreement in the literature so far about the best therapeutic procedure for ovarian cysts. Whereas some authors [9, 28, 36] recommend excision of any diagnosed cyst to avoid complications such as torsion or damage to the bowels, others prefer conservative observation [11, 29]. An argument for the conservative attitude is frequent bilateral appearance of the cysts and frequent spontaneous healing during the first year of life. Treatment with medroxyprogesterone acetate, as recommended by Sedin et al. [29] is indicated for hormone-producing cysts only.

As a rule, we observe endocrine-inactive symptom-free cysts primarily, and we excise only cysts that grow rapidly or that have a primary diameter of more than 5 cm. We have no experience with laparoscopic puncture of the cysts.

Childhood up to Puberty

Two girls with endocrine-active follicular cysts belonged to this group; their medical histories are described here in brief. The girl F. K. was hospitalized at 5 years and 9 months of age for vaginal hemorrhage. Clinical examination revealed slightly feminized external genitalia and markedly enlarged breasts. A vaginal smear showed estrogen-stimulated epithelial cells. E2 was elevated, at 36 pmol/l. Autonomous ovarian estrogen production could be deduced from the missing increase of LH and FHS following LHRH stimulation. Ultrasonographically and radiologically, a cystic tumor was found in the left pelvis; it could not be unequivocally appointed to the left ovary. On laparotomy, an ovarian cyst measuring 6 cm in diameter was found. No ovarian tissue was visible macroscopically, so the cyst was removed in toto. The right ovary appeared macroscopically normal. Pathohistological examination disclosed a follicular cyst. Serum estradiol levels (E2, 3 pmol/l) dropped to normal within 1 week after surgery.

The girl R. S. was admitted to hospital at the age of 3.5 years because of an enlarged clitoris. Serum estrogens were normal. However, serum testosterone and dehydroepiandrostenone were clearly elevated. Laparoscopy revealed several small cysts in both ovaries. These were removed during subsequent laparotomy, but the ovaries were preserved. Pathohistological examination revealed follicular cysts. Testosterone and dehydroepiandrostenone levels normalized within 1 week after surgery. However, the size of the clitoris remained unchanged.

Follicular cysts are frequently found in girls with premature signs of puberty. There is no general agreement in the literature regarding therapeutic procedures, since on the one hand, the cysts may disappear spontaneously; on the other hand, a granulosa cell tumor may be the cause of premature puberty. Kosloske et al. [17], for instance, recommend excision of the cysts, since they observed rapid disappearance of the signs of puberty in their two patients following surgery. Lyon et al. [23] performed cystectomy twice and conservative observation seven times in nine girls with pubertas praecox and ovarian cysts. The conservatively observed cysts all disappeared. Lightner and Kelch [22] and Stanhope and Brook [30] recommend a conservative attitude with cysts less than 3 cm in diameter. The reason for surgical treatment of our patient with an estrogen-producing ovarian cyst was its size. In our patient with androgen-producing cysts, the cysts were enucleated from the ovaries and the serum hormone levels normalized rapidly. In a parallel case [24] similar cysts were simply observed for a longer period of time. Hormone levels finally normalized and the signs of puberty disappeared in this case as well. We are of the opinion that a conservative attitude is justified with cysts less than 5 cm in diameter, since the granulosa cell tumor is extraordinarily rare in this age-group [18, 27]. An active procedure becomes necessary, however, if signs of puberty increase and the cysts are enlarged at ultrasound follow-up.

Post-menarche

Eleven of the 15 girls with follicular cysts (75%) belonged to this age-group. Acute abdominal pain led to hospitalization in all cases. It is not surprising that acute appendicitis was usually the suspected diagnosis, because ten ovarian cysts were located on the right side. No cyst exhibited autonomous hormone production. Follicular cysts which contained up to 200 ml fluid were surgically enucleated and the ovarian tissue was sutured. Like Scheye et al. [26], we recommend excision of cysts larger than 5 cm, also because of the differential diagnosis of a granulosa cell tumor, which is not so rare in this age-group.

Paraovarian Cysts

Paraovarian cysts originate from the epoophoron and are located in the mesosalpinx. Although they do not stem from ovarian tissue, they are mentioned here because they occur close to the ovary. Our five girls were 11–16 years of age and post menarche. Ultrasonographically and radiologically, paraovarian cysts were indistinguishable from ovarian follicular cysts. On laparotomy, the largest paraovarian cyst contained as much as 2 l of fluid. The cysts were enucleated from the mesosalpinx in such a way that the fallopian tube and ovary were not damaged. All patients are well postoperatively without evidence of recurrence.

Conclusion

We recommend the following procedure if an ovarian tumor is suspected: radiological and ultrasonographical examination to determine side and extent of the tumor and sampling of AFP and HCG, as well as of serum estrogens in girls who have not reached puberty. A unilateral ovariectomy is carried out for benign ovarian tumors; organ preservation is rarely possible. With cystic ovarian tumors up to 5 cm in diameter a conservative approach may be employed, with frequent clinical and radiological follow-ups. In all other cases laparotomy is advisable, possibly following laparoscopy. The aim of surgery is to preserve as much of the organ as possible. For malignant tumors a unilateral salpingo-oophorectomy is carried out. Intraoperative staging is supported by peritoneal cytology. Postoperative treatment depends on the histological diagnosis and the extent of the tumor. Curative treatment is possible even if the tumor already extends beyond the organ borders. Levi et al. [21] reported on 253 patients with advanced malignant ovarian tumors. Cure was achieved in 68% by means of a chemotherapeutic regimen also used by us (cisplatin, vinblastine, and bleomycin). To date second-look laparotomy is not recommended [6, 25] and we have not yet performed it, particularly as small recurrent tumors can be diagnosed early by ultrasound. If the surgeon encounters a pathological finding of the ovaries during an appendectomy, the incision should be enlarged to provide a good view of the ovaries. Further treatment should be decided on by an interdisciplinary group consisting of the pediatric surgeon, an endocrinologist, a pediatric gynecologist, and an oncologist.

References

1. Adelman S, Benson CD, Hertzler JH (1975) Surgical lesions of the ovary in infancy and childhood. Surg Gynecol Obstet 141:219–222
2. Adkins JC (1986) Malignant ovarian and other germ cell tumors. In: Hays DM (ed) Pediatric surgical oncology. Grune and Stratton, Orlando, pp 123–138
3. Benz J (1987) Die Früherkennung bösartiger Tumoren in der Gynäkologie. Swiss Med 9/4: 31–43
4. Billmire DF, Grosfeld JL (1986) Teratomas in childhood: analysis of 142 cases. J Pediatr Surg 21:548–551
5. Breen JL, Maxson WS (1977) Ovarian tumors in children and adolescents. Clin Obstet Gynecol 20:607–623
6. Chambers SK, Chambers JT, Kohorn EI, Lawrence R, Schwartz PE (1988) Evaluation of the role of second-look surgery in ovarian cancer. Obstet Gynecol 72:404–408
7. Cronen PW, Nagaraj HS (1988) Ovarian tumors in children. South Med J 81:464–468
8. Ehren IM, Mahour GH, Isaacs H (1984) Benign and malignant ovarian tumors in children and adolescents. A review of 63 cases. Am J Surg 147:339–344
9. Frémond B, Guibert L, Jouan H, Milon J, Tekou H, Duval JM, Babut JM (1986) Les kystes de l'ovaire à diagnostic anténatal. Chir Pediatr 27:128–133
10. Gallion HH, Nagell JR van, Donaldson ES, Powell DE (1988) Ovarian dysgerminoma: report of seven cases and review of the literature. Am J Obstet Gynecol 158:591–595
11. Gaudin J, Le Treguilly C, Parent P, Le Guern H, Chabaud JJ, Boog G, Jehannin B (1988) Neonatal ovarian cysts. Twelve cysts with antenatal diagnosis. Pediatr Surg Int 3:158–164

12. Genton CY (1983) Histopathologie des weiblichen Genitaltraktes. Springer, Berlin Heidelberg New York
13. Giacoia GP, Wood BP (1987) Radiological case of the month. Am J Dis Child 141:1005–1006
14. Grob M (1957) Lehrbuch der Kinderchirurgie. Thieme, Stuttgart, p 133
15. Groeber WR (1963) Ovarian tumors during infancy and childhood. Am J Obstet Gynecol 86:1027–1035
16. Käser O, Friedberg V, Ober KG, Thomsen IK, Zandler J (1969) Gynäkologie und Geburtshilfe, vol 1. Thieme, Stuttgart, pp 232–249
17. Kosloske Am, Goldthorn JF, Kaufman E, Hayek A (1984) Treatment of precocious pseudopuberty associated with follicular cysts of the ovary. Am J Dis Child 138:147–149
18. Kurman RJ, Norris HJ (1976) Endodermal sinus tumor of the ovary, a clinical and pathologic analysis of 71 cases. Cancer 38:2402–2419
19. Lacson AG, Gillis DA, Shawwa A (1988) Malignant mixed germ-cell-sex-cord-stromal tumors of the ovary associated with isosexual precocious puberty. Cancer 61:2122–2133
20. La Vecchia C, Morris HB, Draper GJ (1983) Malignant ovarian tumours in childhood in Britain, 1962–1978. B J Cancer 48:363–374
21. Levi JA. Thomson D, Sandman T, Tattersall M, Raghavan D, Byrne M, Gill G, Harvey V, Burns I, Snyder R (1988) A prospective study of cisplatin-based combination chemotherapy in advanced germ cell malignancy: role of maintenance and long-term follow-up. J Clin Oncol 6:1154–1160
22. Lightner ES, Kelch RP (1984) Treatment of precocious pseudopuberty associated with ovarian cysts. Am J Dis Child 138:126–128
23. Lyon AJ, De Bruyn R, Grant DB (1985) Transient sexual precocity and ovarian cysts. Arch Dis Child 60:819–822
24. Muritano M, Zachmann M, Manella M, Briner J, Prader A (1987) Transient ovarian testosterone and androstenedione hypersecretion: a cause of virilization or premature pubarche in prepubertal girls. Horm Res 28:37–41
25. Pippit CH, Cain JM, Hakes TB, Pierce VK, Lewis JL (1988) Primary chemotherapy and the role of second-look laparotomy in non-dysgerminomatous germ cell malignancies of the ovary. Gynecol Oncol 31:268–275
26. Scheye T, Rodier JF, Vannenville G, Souteyrand P, Dechelotte P, Billet P, Lesec G, Vorilhou P (1986) Kystes bénins de l'ovaire. Expérience homogène de 22 cas receuillis en 10 ans. Chir Pediatr 27:185–189
27. Schneider A (1983) Granulosa cell tumour in a child. Prog Pediatr Surg 16:127–132
28. Scholz PM, Key L, Filston HC (1982) Large ovarian cyst causing cecal perforation in a newborn infant. J Pediatr Surg 17:91–92
29. Sedin G, Bergquist C, Lindgren PG (1985) Ovarian hyperstimulation syndrome in preterm infants. Pediatr Res 19:548–552
30. Stanhope R, Brook CGD (1985) Precocious pseudopuberty and ovarian follicular cysts. Am J Dis Child 139:222
31. Steck AM (1954) Les tumeurs ovariennes chez l'enfant. Helv Paediat Acta 9:69–87
32. Towne BH, Mahour GH, Wooley MM, Isaacs H (1975) Ovarian cysts and tumors in infancy and childhood. J Pediatr Surg 10:311–320
33. Trenner J, Niethammer D, Schweizer P, Fischbach H, Flach A (1983) Malignant ovarian tumours during childhood. Prog Pediatr Surg 16:121–126
34. Vassal G, Flamant F, Caillaud JM, Demeocq F, Nihoul Fékété C, Lemerle J (1988) Juvenile granulosa cell tumor of the ovary in children: a clinical study of 15 cases. J Clin Oncol 6:990–995
35. Weinblatt ME, Ortega JA (1982) Treatment of children with dysgerminoma of the ovary. Cancer 49:2608–2611
36. Zachariou Z, Roth H, Daum R, Schmidt W, Hofmann W, Hauf-Zachariou U (1987) Ovarialpseudocysten bei weiblichen Neugeborenen: pränatale ultrasonographische Diagnose und chirurgische Konsequenz. Z Kinderchir 42:126–130

Recent Developments
in the Management of Neuroblastoma

M. L. Nieder and M. W. L. Gauderer

Summary

Neuroblastoma was first described in 1864 by Virchow [44]. For the next 100 years, the primary approach to these patients was predominantly surgical resection. With the advent of multimodal adjuvant treatments using chemotherapy and irradiation in the 1950s and 1960s, coordination of multispecialty therapeutic interventions became important. By the late 1970s, effective neoadjuvant chemotherapeutic regimens enabled some inoperable tumors to be completely removed at the time of "second look" procedures. In the 1980s, advances in tumor biology and imaging gave new insight and novel prognostic indicators which helped determine the course of therapy. In the 1990s, treating poor risk patients with extremely high dose chemotherapy, irradiation, and allogeneic or autologous bone marrow rescue with or without surgical resection may finally improve the survival of these children.

Zusammenfassung

Das Neuroblastom wurde erstmalig im Jahr 1864 von Virchow beschrieben. Während der nächsten hundert Jahre wurde die chirurgische Resektion als alleinige Therapie der Wahl davon betroffenen Patienten angesehen. Mit der Entwicklung multimodaler, adjuvanter Therapiemethoden wie Bestrahlung oder Chemotherapie in den 50er und 60er Jahren gewann die Koordination interdisziplinärer Behandlungskonzepte immer mehr an Bedeutung. Seit den späten 70er Jahren ermöglichen effektive adjuvante Chemotherapieprotokolle die komplette Entfernung ursprünglich inoperabler Tumoren in einer "second-look-Operation". In den 80er Jahren ergaben Fortschritte in der Tumorbiologie sowie der Tumordarstellung neue Gesichtspunkte und neue prognostische Marker, die zur Festlegung des Therapieverlaufs beitrugen. In den 90er Jahren wird möglicherweise die Behandlung von Patienten mit schlechter Prognose durch extrem hohe Chemotherapie, Bestrahlung oder allogene bzw. autologe Knochenmarkstransplantation mit oder ohne chirurgische Intervention endlich zu einer Verbesserung der Heilungschancen führen.

Résumé

Le neuroblastome a été décrit pour la première fois en 1864 par Virchow. Au siècle suivant, le traitement de choix consistait, dans la grande majorité des cas, en une résection chirurgicale. Des thérapeutiques d'appoint telles que chimiothérapie et radiothérapie ayant fait leur apparition pendant les années 50 et 60, il est devenu indispensable de bien coordonner ces thérapeutiques relevant de spécialisations multiples. Vers la fin des années 70, la chimiothérapie adjuvante permit de faire disparaître certaines tumeurs par une intervention dite de "second look" inopérables

---

Divisions of Pediatric Hematology/Oncology and Pediatric Surgery Rainbow Babies' and Children's Hospital and Case Western Reserve University School of Medicine, 2074 Abington Road, Cleveland, OH 44106, USA.

Progress in Pediatric Surgery, Vol. 26
Gauderer and Angerpointner (Eds.)
© Springer-Verlag Berlin Heidelberg 1991

à l'origine. Durant les années 80, les progrès réalisés en biologie et en imagerie dans le domaine des tumeurs permirent de déterminer de nouveaux facteurs donnant la possibilité de prévoir l'évolution et l'issue de la maladie et d'en organiser le traitement en conséquence. Au cours des années 90, il sera peut-être possible de prolonger la survie des enfants ayant un pronostic très défavorable en ayant recours à la chimiothérapie à dose très élevée, à la radiothérapie, à la transplantation autologue ou allogénique de moelle osseuse, avec ou sans résection chirurgicale.

Introduction

Neuroblastoma affects young children and comprises almost 50% of the malignancies among infants [7]. It is the third most common solid tumor in children aged 1–15 years and is usually widespread at the time of diagnosis [29]. In more than 50% of cases, the abdomen is the site of the primary tumor [29]. Because the tumor is of neural crest origin, primary sites have been reported in every location which has sympathetic nerve innervation [33]. Though prognosis was once solely linked to age and stage of disease, recent advances in molecular biology have afforded a better understanding of the biologic basis of this disease.

Pathologic Diagnosis

Since the diagnosis of neuroblastoma cannot always be made on morphologic characteristics, immunophenotyping can assist the pathologist in distinguishing between neuroblastoma, leukemia, lymphoma, rhabdomyosarcoma, and Ewing's sarcoma. The success of immunophenotyping rests on the sensitivity and specificity of the monoclonal antibodies. Monoclonal antibodies now used for the immunophenotyping of leukemia and lymphoma are quite specific and can usually differentiate these entities from neuroblastoma. Similarly, immunoperoxidase staining can identify muscle-associated tumors like rhabdomyosarcoma. Neuron-specific enolase, once thought to be helpful in identifying neuroblastoma, has unfortunately proven to be problematic [12]. Other monoclonal antibodies such as HSAN 1.2 [41], GD2, HNK.1, and HLA are now being used in the diagnostic workup of the tumor [43]. The combined use of these monoclonals will give a pattern of results which contribute to the final pathologic diagnosis. However, distinguishing neuroblastoma from primitive neural ectodermal tumors continues to be difficult [43].

Biologic Characteristics

Neuroblastoma is considered to be part of the APUD (amine precursor uptake decarboxylse) group of tumors. These neural crest tumors synthesize and secrete adrenergic catecholamines such as homovanillic acid (HVA), vanillylmandelic acid (VMA), and vanillacetic acid. Though Laug et al. [31] demonstrated that the specific catecholamine metabolite was not of prognostic significance, they noted that a low VMA:HVA ratio may indicate poor outcome. This phenomenon may be related to the aggressive nature of those tumors which lack dopamine beta-hydroxylase (and hence cannot produce VMA from HVA).

Cytogenetic studies of actual neuroblastoma tissue specimens have revealed chromosomal abnormalities in approximately 80% of cases [4]. Most of these abnormalities involve the short arm of chromosome 1 [6]. Interestingly, unlike the majority of solid tumors which affect adults, tumor cell hyperdiploidy (increased DNA content) has been associated with a better prognosis [18, 32]. Results of neuroblastoma tumor cell cycle analysis (proliferative activity) suggest that more rapidly dividing tumors may portend a worse prognosis [10]. In addition to tumor cell kinetics, Northern and Southern blotting techniques have revealed that patients with poor prognosis neuroblastoma have increased numbers of the N-*myc* oncogene in the tumor genome as well as excess N-*myc* messenger RNA (mRNA) in tumor cells [38, 39].

The oncogene N-*myc* is normally found on chromosome 2, but is translocated to chromosome 1 and amplified in some cases of neuroblastoma. N-*myc* is amplified (increased numbers of gene copies) or overexpressed (increased mRNA or N-*myc* protein) in half the patients with stage III or IV disease [39]. Patients with stage I, II, or IVS disease rarely show tumor cell N-*myc* amplification or overexpression [8, 39]. N-*myc* amplification studies are important components of the evaluation of a child with neuroblastoma. The prognostic significance of N-*myc* gene copy number has been recognized and these results are now being used as part of the eligibility criteria in Children's Cancer Study Group neuroblastoma studies (CCSG study 3881).

Other prognostic indicators include serum ferritin values (elevated in some poor-prognosis patients), serum neuron-specific enolase (elevated in some poor-prognosis patients), age and stage of the patient at diagnosis, and location of the tumor [29, 30]. Though multivariate analysis has determined that most of these biochemical aberrations may not be independently significant, biochemical markers do prove useful when following the clinical status and progress of treatment in these children.

An especially favorable prognosis is conferred upon those two percent of patients who present with ataxia and opsomyoclonus accompanying their neuroblastoma [1, 3, 9]. Unfortunately, the neurological sequelae often persist even when the child is free of disease. In addition to those patients who present with opsomyoclonus, those few patients with ganglioneuroblastoma and diarrhea caused by secretion of vasoactive intestinal polypeptides also have a favorable outcome [11, 13, 28]. In contrast to the patients with opsomyoclonus, children with diarrhea become asymptomatic after the tumor is removed.

Tumor Imaging

Assessment of the clinical status of tumors in children advanced significantly in the 1980s. The improvements in computer software resulted in outstanding image quality with computed tomography (CT). The emergence of magnetic resonance imaging (MRI) as a distinct modality within radiology has led to better studies of certain organs and soft tissue. Advances in nuclear medicine made meta-iodo-benzylguanidine (MIBG) scanning an important diagnostic tool in many centers [27, 36]. Though still experimental, immunolocalization of neuroblastoma using radiolabeled monoclonal antibodies and gamma scanning began in the 1980's and is being used in some centers today [7, 20]. MIBG and monoclonal antibody-mediated nuclear scanning can identify some small tumors which go unnoticed on CT, MRI, or conventional nuclear medicine scans. Localization of small residual tumors is now possible and can help determine which children are candidates for further surgical procedures.

Surgical Management

Operative techniques and anesthesia have improved significantly over the past several decades, Therefore, localized tumors should be removed in an attempt to eliminate all gross disease. In those cases where less than 90% of the tumor can be resected, only a biopsy should be performed. Those patients with residual disease will undergo chemotherapy in an attempt to substantially reduce the size of the tumor.

Patients with residual disease whose tumor responds favorably to chemotherapy are good candidates for aggressive "second look" surgical procedures [16, 24]. The removal of all gross tumor prior to consolidation, maintenance, or ablative chemotherapy and radiotherapy is thought to enhance the possibility of prolonged disease-free survival [24].

Supportive Care

Beside the technological strides made over the past 20 years, supportive care techniques have improved the quality of life for children with cancer. Insertion of central venous access devices has minimized the possibility of chemotherapy extravasation as well as making treatment and diagnostic sessions less uncomfortable [19]. The ease of vascular access has eliminated the single greatest cause of fear in these children undergoing cancer treatment. The medical and nursing expertise in dealing with critically ill children has ripened and pediatric intensive care units now provide outstanding care. The improved outcome of many patients with neuroblastoma is related not only to nuances in therapy but also to a better understanding of the well-being of the whole child. The cooperation between physicians, nurses, child life specialists, psychologists, and social workers has resulted in excellent comprehensive treatment for children and their families.

Patients

From January, 1975 to December, 1989, 100 children with neuroblastoma were treated at Rainbow Babies' and Children's Hospital in Cleveland, Ohio. The initial staging data on these patients were similar to hose reported in other large studies and within the CCSG: stage I, 14%; stage II, 15%; stage III, 18%; stage IV, 41%; stage IV-S, 12%. During this period, the children were treated with a variety of multiagent chemotherapeutic regimens. Those patients with advanced or relapsed disease were enrolled in pilot studies using high-dose chemotherapy and bone marrow rescue. Because of the variation in treatment over the years, it is not feasible to report outcome data even on this large group of patients.

Treatment

A multidisciplinary approach to the patient with neuroblastoma is mandatory for optimal outcome. A complete surgical resection of the tumor at the time of diagnosis is clearly the treatment of choice. However, when such a resection is impossible or when distant metastases are present, initial tumor control by chemotherapy and/or radiotherapy is necessary. Since the ultimate prognosis is not based on age and stage alone, a portion of the tumor should be submitted for bio-

Table 1. Evans staging system for neuroblastoma

Stage	Criteria
Stage I	Tumor confined to the organ or structure of origin
Stage II	Tumor extending in continuity beyond the organ or structure of origin but not crossing the midline. Regional lymph nodes on the homolateral side may be involved
Stage III	Tumors extending in continuity beyond the midline. Regional lymph nodes bilaterally may be involved
Stage IV	Remote disease involving bone, parenchymatous organs, soft tissues or distant lymph node groups, or bone marrow
Stage IV-S	Patients who would otherwise be stage I or II but who have remote disease confined to one or more of the following sites: liver, skin, or bone marrow (without evidence of bone metastases)

Table 2. Pediatric Oncology Group staging for neuroblastoma

Stage	Criteria
Stage A	Complete gross excision of primary tumor, margins histologically negative or positive. Intracavitary lymph nodes not intimately adhered to and removed with resected tumor are histologically free of tumor. If primary is in abdomen (including pelvis), liver is histologically free of tumor
Stage B	Incomplete gross resection of primary. Lymph nodes and liver histologically free of tumor as in Stage A
Stage C	Complete or incomplete gross resection of primary. Intracavitary nodes histologically positive for tumor. Liver histologically free of tumor
Stage D	Disseminated disease beyond intracavitary nodes (i.e., bone marrow, bone, liver, skin, or lymph nodes beyond cavity containing primary tumor)

chemical and molecular biological analysis. If such analysis is not readily available, a portion of the tumor should be quickly frozen for future testing.

Presently, the staging of neuroblastoma is based on two different systems (Tables 1, 2). The St. Jude Children's Research Hospital staging method adopted by the Pediatric Oncology Group (POG) is dependent upon surgical-pathologic criteria, while the Evans staging method used by the CCSG relies on physical examination, imaging studies, and bone marrow aspiration/biopsy [14, 26]. In the future, a staging system encompassing both clinical and molecular biology parameters will be more useful. Regardless of the staging system, the following guidelines should be considered when treating patients with neuroblastoma:

Resectable Tumors Without Metastases

A gross total surgical resection should be attempted. As in all initial surgical procedures in patients suspected of having neuroblastoma, excision of adjacent organs is not indicated. However, if a para-aortic primary tumor invades the renal vessels, radical nephrectomy may be performed. If the primary tumor cannot be completely removed, surgical debulking should be attempted only if 90%–95% of the mass can be excised.

Those patients with complete resections and negative lymph nodes are not candidates for chemotherapy or radiotherapy. If the entire tumor was not resected or if pathological examination demonstrates lymph node spread, further therapy may be recommended. However, Matthay and colleagues [34] reported that chemotherapy and/or radiotherapy in stage II patients did not improve survival. To identify a subgroup of stage II patients who might benefit from additional treatment, N-*myc* amplification results are being used in some studies as the determining factor for further chemotherapy (CCSG 3881). In other settings, these children have received local radiotherapy or short-term multiagent chemotherapy [22].

Resectable Tumors with Limited Metastatic Spread

The care of patients with localized metastatic disease (e.g., involved lymph nodes) has garnered controversy over the past decade. In the Evans staging system, these patients are classified as either stage III or IV-S (special). The approach to these children has been age-related, since younger children historically have fared better [29, 30]. Young infants with abdominal primary tumors may have respiratory distress, and a resection of the tumor mass may have immediate therapeutic value. Even if the tumor cannot be resected, biopsy alone followed by insertion of an abdominal wall extender (patch or silo) may be beneficial [15]. Though surgical resection of the primary tumor may have been achieved, extensive procedures to remove all areas of metastases should not be employed. In patients presenting with the syndrome of ataxia and opsomyoclonus, excellent outcomes are achieved with surgical resection alone [1, 3].

Some infants with stage IV-S or stage C/D disease receive chemotherapy with or without radiotherapy [22]. While some of these babies had spontaneous regression of their disease, those that did usually had small primary tumors and no bone marrow involvement [15]. There is evidence to suggest that infants whose tumor exhibits no N-*myc* amplification will do well without either chemotherapy or radiotherapy, and the current CCSG study recommends no therapy for these patients (CCSG study 3881). In this study, infants in this group whose tumor cells have N-*myc* amplification will receive multiagent chemotherapy. Other strategy groups recommend a short course of chemotherapy with limited agents, and additional drugs such as *cis*-platinum should be used only if remission is not achieved early [22].

The treatment of older children with limited metastatic disease (e.g., lymph nodes) should include chemotherapy with or without radiotherapy. In some aggressive protocols, radiotherapy is reserved as a local control measure in patients with unresectable disease after chemotherapy. Since investigators have reported a poor outcome in patients with tumor cell N-*myc* amplification, those patients should receive extensive chemotherapy [6, 38, 39]. Additional treatment with high dose chemotherapy and bone marrow rescue should be considered in those individuals with N-*myc* amplification within the tumor cells [40].

Resectable and Nonresectable Primary Tumors with Widespread Metastases

In the majority of these cases, the diagnosis can be made by bone marrow aspiration and urinary catecholamine elevation. However, it is extremely important to obtain an adequate specimen for tumor cell studies, and a tissue biopsy may be necessary to achieve this. There are very few cases where an extensive primary surgical procedure can be justified in cases of widespread metastatic disease. Children with evidence of metastatic disease should have a primary surgical debulking only if the diagnosis cannot be confirmed by a less invasive procedure.

All such patients receive multiagent chemotherapy with the intent of significantly decreasing the size of the primary tumor and alleviating metastatic spread. Children who enjoy a good response to chemotherapy are then ideal candidates for delayed surgical procedures. The goal of delayed surgical intervention is to assess the effect of therapy and remove any gross residual disease [16, 24]. Following this, further chemotherapy, radiotherapy, or high dose chemotherapy with bone marrow rescue may be used. A few institutions are studying the therapeutic efficacy of cytotoxic agents linked to neuroblastoma-seeking monoclonal antibodies in an effort to eliminate minimal residual disease [7]. This is used in addition to systemic chemotherapy.

Discussion

Until recently, the survival of children with widespread neuroblastoma had not changed since the early 1960s. Although a multimodal approach had been coordinated with surgery, irradiation, and chemotherapy, initially responsive tumors would usually recur after therapy ceased [25]. Thus, children were living longer but their ultimate survival was not affected.

In the latter part of the 1980s, improvements in bone marrow transplantation techniques led to the development of better conditioning regimens [37, 40]. As such, residual tumor can be eliminated without lethal toxicity. The use of bone marrow transplantation as consolidation therapy early in the course of the disease may one day be the treatment of choice for patients with widespread neuroblastoma. If results of autologous bone marrow rescue using monoclonal antibody-purged bone marrow continue to be similar to these obtained with allogeneic rescue, then the morbidity and mortality of graft-versus-host disease can be eliminated by autologous transplantation techniques [21, 40].

In addition to the severe financial constraints, bone marrow transplantation is an intensive undertaking fraught with significant toxicities. Bone marrow transplantation as consolidation therapy should be considered only when clinical and molecular biological data have been assessed. N-*myc* oncogene amplification in tumor cells of patients with stage I, II, III, and IV-S disease confers a poor prognosis; these patients should be given intensive therapy. Since patients with stage IV disease have such a poor prognosis, N-*myc* analysis cannot be used as a prognostic indicator in such cases.

Some patients with recurrent disease have exhibited tumor responses to infusions of monoclonal antibodies which can bind to receptors on neuroblastoma cells [7]. This investigational therapy has been performed in a limited number of institutions and long-term followup is presently not available. In the 1990s, in vivo monoclonal antibody infusions may be incorporated into chemotherapeutic regimens, will be used in nuclear imaging techniques, and could become an additional part of the conditioning regimens for bone marrow transplantation.

Patients with advanced disease who are candidates for bone marrow transplantation will benefit from the use of growth factor infusions. Results from adult studies in the 1980s suggest that duration of neutropenia can be reduced with growth factors, thus lessening the risk of sepsis [2]. Growth factor infusions are also being used with experimental chemotherapy protocols to reduce marrow recovery time, decrease the incidence of infection, and increase the frequency of therapy [23]. Since the main problem with neuroblastoma treatment has been one of recurrent disease, intensifying therapy may be beneficial until superior drug regimens are available. Drug resistance of tumor cells, another major dilemma of treatment, is being addressed as more studies on the multidrug resistance gene and P-glycoprotein are undertaken [35].

The diagnosis, treatment, and management of patients with neuroblastoma has become extremely complex. It is imperative that all newly diagnosed patients undergo a thorough evaluation. Each workup should include appropriate imaging studies, pathology review, serum and urine studies, molecular biology analysis of tumor cells and tumor marker analysis. In the 1990s, optimal therapeutic intervention should be based on results of all the aforementioned tests. Therefore, the care of children with neuroblastoma should be rendered in large children's hospitals and centers with pediatric oncology expertise. The children's hospital in the 1990s also provides comprehensive psychosocial support to patients and their families which cannot be given elsewhere. Such support is of equal importance to medical care in the treatment of these children. Finally, our knowledge of the pathophysiology of this disease will grow only when patients are enrolled in groupwide studies, receive standardized treatment, and are managed by a compassionate team approach.

Illustrative Case

A 15-month-old white female presented with pronounced abdominal distention, pallor, and irritability. Imaging studies revealed a huge mass occupying the entire

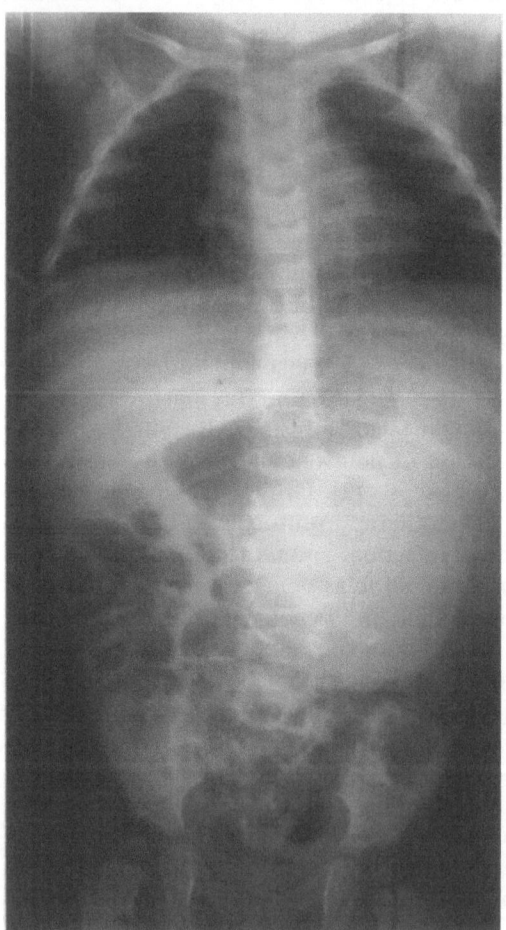

Fig. 1. Abdominal radiograph of a 15-month-old child with neuroblastoma. A large abdominal mass which elevates the diaphragm and displaces the bowel caudally can be identified. Note the presence of calcification within the tumor and the partial destruction of the left 12th rib

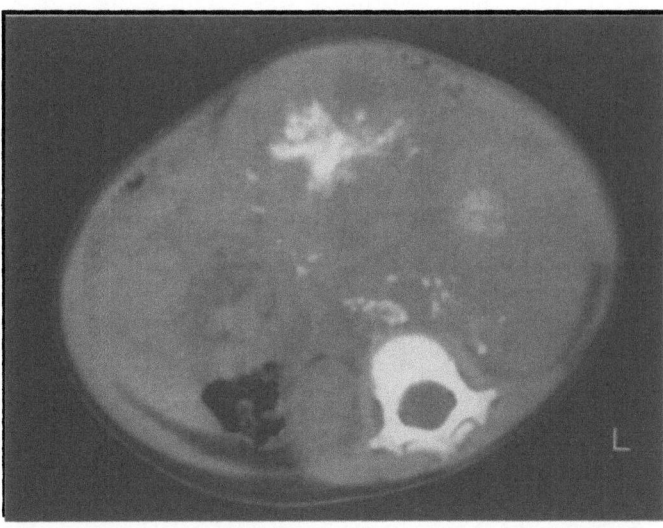

Fig. 2. Computed tomogram of the upper abdomen demonstrating the massive size of the partially calcified tumor. Because of the tumor size and location, it was initially assessed as being unresectable

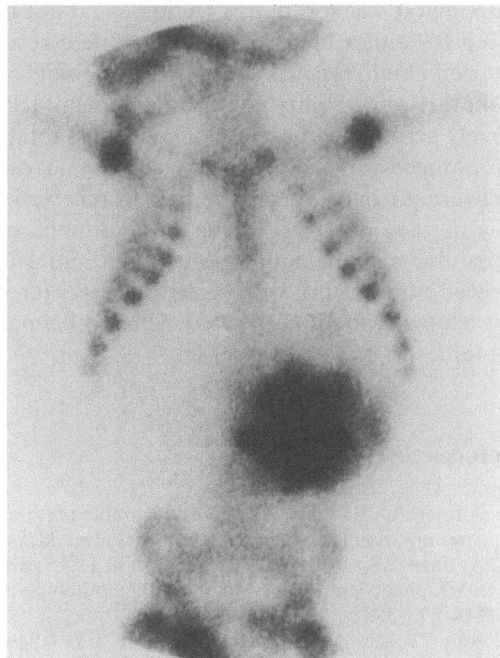

Fig. 3. Technetium-99m MDP total body bone scan showing intense uptake within the tumor

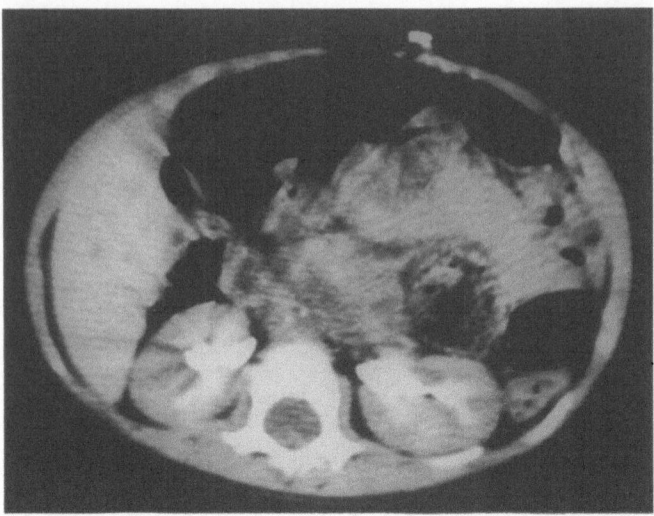

Fig. 4. Computed tomography 9 months after gross total resection reveals no evidence of residual disease. Both kidneys appear normal and demonstrate appropriate excretion of contrast material

upper abdomen with destruction of a portion of her left 12th rib (Figs. 1–3). Although it was felt that resection could not be accomplished, the child was prepared for either biopsy only or complete resection. Reexamination of the anesthetized child revealed some tumor mobility. A small incision was initially made and after resectability could be demonstrated, the incision was extended transversely across the upper abdomen. Gross total tumor resection was achieved after a prolonged surgical procedure. Bone marrow examinations were normal. After recovering from surgery, the patient received 11 cycles of multiagent chemotherapy in the next year using *cis*-platinum, cyclophosphamide, etoposide, and doxorubicin. Nine months after her initial diagnosis, her abdominal CT scan showed no evidence of disease (Fig. 4). Her initial serum ferritin and tumor N-*myc* studies were not elevated. She has been off chemotherapy for 9 months and continues to be free of disease.

References

1. Altman AJ, Baehner RL (1976) Favorable prognosis for survival in children with coincident opso-myoclonus and neuroblastoma. Cancer 37:846–852
2. Antman KS, Griffin JD, Elias A, et al (1988) Effect of recombinant human granulocyte-macrophage stimulating factor on chemotherapy-induced myelosuppression. N Engl J Med 319:593–598
3. Bray PF, Ziter FA, Lahey ME, Myers GG (1969) The coincidence of neuroblastoma and cerebellar encephalopathy. J Pediatr 75:983–990
4. Brodeur GM, Sekhon GS, Goldstein MN (1977) Chromosomal aberrations in human neuroblastomas. Cancer 40:2256–2263

5. Brodeur GM, Seeger RC, Schwab M, Varmus HE, Bishop JM (1984) Amplification of N-*myc* in untreated human neuroblastomas correlates with advanced disease stage. Science 224:1121–1124

6. Brodeur GM, Font CT, Morita M, et al (1988) Molecular analysis and clinical significance of N-*myc* amplification and chromosomal 1p monosomy in human neuroblastomas. Prog Clin Biol Res 271:3–15

7. Cheung NK, Saarinen U, Neely J, et al (1985) Monoclonal antibodies to a glycolipid antigen on human neuroblastoma cells. Cancer Res 45:2642–2649

8. Christiansen H, Lampert F (1988) Tumour karyotype discriminates between good and bad prognostic outcome in neuroblastoma. Br J Cancer 57:121–126

9. Cohn SL, Salwen H, Herst CV, Maurer HS, Nieder ML, Morgan ER, Rosen ST (1988) Single copies of the N-*myc* oncogene in neuroblastomas from children presenting with the syndrome of opsoclonus-myoclonus. Cancer 62:723–726

10. Cohn SL, Rademaker AW, Salwen HR, et al (1990) Analysis of DNA ploidy and proliferative activity in relation to histology and N-*myc* amplification in neuroblastoma. Am J Pathol

11. Cooney DR, Vorhees ML, Fisher JE (1982) Vasoactive intestinal polypeptide-producing neuroblastoma. J Pediatr Surg 17:821

12. Dranoff G, Bigner DD (1984) A word of caution to the use of neuron-specific enolase expression in tumor diagnosis (editorial). Arch Path Lab Med 108:535

13. El-Shafie M, Samule D, Klippel CH (1983) Intractable diarrhea in children with VIP-secreting ganglioneuroblastoma. J Pediatr Surg 18:34

14. Evans AE, D'Angio GJ, Randolf J (1971) A proposed staging system for children with neuroblastoma. Cancer 27:374–378

15. Evans AE, Chatten J, D'Angio GJ, et al (1980) A review of 17 IV-S neuroblastoma patients at the Children's Hospital of Philadelphia. Cancer 45:833–839

16. Exelby PR (1984) Pediatric oncology surgery. In: Sutow WW, Fernbach DJ, Vietti TJ (eds) Clinical pediatric oncology, 3rd edn. Mosby, St Louis, pp 154–166

17. Gale G, D'Angio G, Uri A, Chatten J, Koop CE (1982) Cancer in neonates: the experience at the Children's Hospital of Philadelphia. Pediatrics 70:409–413

18. Gansler T, Chatten J, Varello M, Bunin G, Atkinson B (1986) Flow cytometric analysis of neuroblastoma: Cancer 58:2453–2458

19. Gauderer MWL, Stellato TA (1985) Subclavin broviac catheters in children: technical considerations in 146 placements. J Pediatr Surg 20 (4):402–405

20. Goldman A, Vivian G, Gordon I, et al (1984) Immunolocalization of neuroblastoma using radiolabeled monoclonal antibody UJ13A. J Pediatr 105:252–256

21. Graham-Pole J (1989) Magnetic antibody technique improves survival in neuroblastoma. Biotechnol Oncol News 3(12):1

22. Green AA, Hayes FA, Hustu HO (1981) Sequential cyclophosphamide and doxorubicin for induction of complete remission in children with disseminated neuroblastoma. Cancer 48:2310–2317

23. Groopman JE, Molina JM, Scadden DT (1989) Hematopoietic growth factors: biology and clinical applications. N Engl J Med 321:1149–1459

24. Grosfeld JL (1986) Neuroblastoma. In: Welch KJ et al (eds) Pediatric surgery, 4th edn. Yearbook Medical, Chicago, pp 283–293

25. Hayes FA, Smith EI (1989) Neuroblastoma. In: Pizzo PA, Poplack DG (eds) Principles and practice of pediatric oncology. Lippincott, Philadelphia, pp 607–622

26. Hayes FA, Green AA, Husto HO, Kumar M (1983) Surgicopathologic staging of neuroblastoma: prognostic significance of regional lymph node metastasis. J Pediatr 102:59–62

27. Hibi S, Todo S, Imashuku S, Miyazaki T (1987) 131-I-Meta-iodobenzylguanidine scintigraphy in patients with neuroblastoma. Pediatr Radiol 17:308–313

28. Jansen-Goemans A, Engelhardt J (1977) Intractable diarrhea in a boy with vasoactive intestinal peptide-producing ganglioneuroblastoma. Pediatrics 59:710–715

29. Jereb B, Bretsky SS, Vogel R, Helson L (1984) Age and prognosis in neuroblastoma. Am J Pediatr Hematol Oncol 6:233–243

30. Kretschmar CS, Frantz CN, Rosen EM, Cassady JR, Levey R, Sallan SE (1984) Improved prognosis for infants with stage IV neuroblastoma. J Clin Oncol 2:799–803
31. Laug WE, Siegel SE, Show KN, et al (1978) Initial urinary catecholamine metabolite concentrations and prognosis in neuroblastoma. Pediatrics 62:77–83
32. Look AT, Hayes FA, Nitschke R, McWilliams NB, Green AA (1984) Cellular DNA content as a predictor of response to chemotherapy in infants with unresectable neuroblastoma. N Engl J Med 311:231–235
33. Machin GA (1982) Histogenesis and histopathology of neuroblastoma. In: Pochedly C (ed) Neuroblastoma: clinical and biological manifestations, Elsevier, New York, pp 194–231
34. Matthay KK, Sather HN, Seeger RC, et al (1989) Excellent outcome of stage II neuroblastoma is independent of residual disease and radiation therapy. J Clin Oncol 7(2):236–244
35. Morrow CS, Cowan KH (1988) Mechanism and clinical significance of multidrug resistance. Oncology 2:55–68
36. Munker T (1985) 131I-Meta-iodobenzylguanidine scintigraphy of neuroblastomas. Semin Nucl Med 15:154–160
37. Reynolds CP, Moss TJ, Feig SA, Selch M, Matthay KK, Wells J, Seeger RC (1989) Treatment of poor prognosis neuroblastoma with intensive therapy and autologous bone marrow transplantation. In: Dicke K, Spitzer G, Jagannath S (eds) Autologous marrow transplantation: proceedings of the fourth international symposium, Houston. University of Texas MD Anderson Hospital and Tumor Institute
38. Rosen N, Reynolds CP, Thiele C, Biedler J, Israel M (1986) Increased N-*myc* expression following progressive growth of human neuroblastoma. Cancer Res 46:4139–4142
39. Seeger RC, Brodeur GM, Sather H, et al (1985) Association of multiple copies of N-*myc* oncogene with rapid progression of neuroblastomas. N Engl J Med 313:1111–1116
40. Seeger RC, Moss TJ, Feig SA, Selch M, Matthay KK, Wells J, Reynolds CP (1989) Autologous bone marrow transplantation for poor prognosis neuroblastoma. In: Champlain R, Gall RP (eds) Bone marrow transplantation: current controversies. Liss, New York, pp 279–288
41. Smith RG, Reynolds CP (1987) Monoclocal antibody recognizing a human neuroblastoma-associated antigen. Diagn Clin Immunol 5:209–220
42. Stephenson S, Cook B, Mease A, Ruymann (1986) The prognostic significance of age and pattern of metastases in stage IV-S neuroblastoma. Cancer 58:372–375
43. Triche TJ (1990) Neuroblastoma and other childhood neural tumors: a review. Pediatr Pathol 10(1–2):175–193
44. Virchow R (1864) Hyperplasie der Zirbel und der Nebennieren. In: Die krankhaften Geschwülste, vol 2. Hirschwald, Berlin

Subject Index

adenocarcinoma, ovarian   115
adenoma
– parathyroid   51
– hyperparathyroidism, primary   51
– thyroid gland   5, 6, 11, 23, 25
– – gland, autonomous   29, 30, 32–35, 37
adenomatosis
– diffuse, PINH   66, 70
– focal, PINH   66, 69, 70
adrenal medullary hyperplasia, pheochromocytoma   106
AFP (alpha-fetoprotein)
– ovarian tumors   116–118
– paraovarian cysts   122
AMPT (alphamethylparathyrosine), pheochromocytoma   109
anaplastic thyroid carcinoma   46
androgen-prodcuing cysts   121
anti-human thyroglobulin   33
anti-microsomal antibody titres   33
anti-thyroid
– antibodies   38
– drug treatment   32
– drugs   32, 37
anti-TSH receptor antibody   33
antibody titres, anti-microsomal   33
APUD (amine precursor uptake decar-
boxylase)
– neuroblastoma   125
– tumors, pheochromocytoma   105
APUD cells, pancreatic head tumor   97
apudoma, pancreatic   97, 98
arteriogram, left renal, pheochromocytoma
   107
autoimmune disease   29
autonomous adenoma
– enucleataion   30
– preoperative thyroid metabolism   30

beta-human-chorionic gonadotropin (beta-
   HCG), ovarian tumors   116–118
blue diaper syndrome   55
bone marrow transplantation, neuroblastoma   131

Braun's anastomosis, pancreatic head tumor
   98

C-cell hyperplasia, familial hyperparathyroidism   53
calcium concentration, parathyroid hormone
   49
cancer (see carcinoma or tumor)
carbimazole   29
carcinoid
– gastrointestinal tract   99, 100
– pancreatic   97, 99
– thyroid (thyroid gland)   5, 6, 11, 16, 18,
   19, 22, 24, 37, 41 ff.
catecholamine
– levels, pheochromocytoma   107, 108
– neuroblastoma   125
CCSG-staging, neuroblastoma   128
cellular immune response, thyroid carcinoma
   42, 44
cervical dissection, thyroid carcinoma   43
chemotherapy
– endodermal sinus tumor   118
– neuroblastoma   127, 128
– – multiagent   130
– ovarian tumors   117
chloride phosphate, parathyroid hormone   50
cholecystojejunostomy, pancreatic head
   tumor   98
cholesterol, serum   32
Cl/P ratio, parathyroid hormone   50
cobalt irradiation, thyroid carcinoma   43
cystadenocarcinoma, ovarian   115
cystadenofibroma, ovarian   115
cystadenoma
– ovarian   115
– serous, ovarian   113
cystadenomas, ovarian   114
cystectomy, ovarian   121
cystic
– ovarian tumors   122
– teratoma, ovarian   116
cyst(s)
– androgen-prodcuing   121

cyst(s)
- corpus luteum, ovarian   113, 119
- dermoid, ovarian   115
- follicular   113, 119, 121
-- endocrine-active   121
- functional, ovarian   115, 119
- ovarian   113, 114
- paraovarian   113–115, 121

DeGeorge's syndrome   57
dermoid cyst, ovarian   115
dextrose, hypertonic, PINH   63
diazoxide
- nesidioblastosis   78
- PINH   63, 65
DNA content, thyroid carcinoma   42
dopamine, pheochromocytoma   108
drugs
- antithyroid   32, 37
- thyrostatic   28, 29
duodenopancratectomy (Whipple procedure)
   96
dysgerminoma, ovarian   113, 117

embryology, thyroid gland   2
endocrine
- adenomatosis, familial   61
-- multiple, types I and II   52
- neoplasia, multiple (MEN), pancreatic
   head tumor   98
-- syndrome, multiple (MEN), type IIb   24
- ophthalmopathy   29, 38
- tumors, gastrointestinal tract   99
-- pancreas   99
endocrine-active tumors, gastrointestinal tract,
   clinical symptoms   100
endocrinopathies
- familial   53
- spontaneous primary hyperparathyroidism   52
endodermal sinus tumor, ovarian (Yolk Sac)
   113–115, 118
enucleation
- nesidioblastosis   89
- ovarian tumors   116
- thyroid carcinoma   37
epinephrine, pheochromocytoma   104, 107
epithelial tumors, ovarian   113, 115
estradiol production, ovarian cysts   120
estrogens, ovarian cysts   119
ethyroidism   34, 35
euglycemia, PINH   63
euthyroid
- nudular goiter   16
- struma   17
Evans staging system, neuroblastoma   128

familial
- endocrine adenomatosis   61
- endocrinopathies   53
- hyperparathyroidism   52ff.
- hypocalciuric hypercalcemia (FHH)   53
fat necrosis, subcutaneous, hyperparathyroidism   55
fetal islet cell formation, nesidioblastosis   92
FHH, familial hypocalciuric hypercalcemia
   53
follicular
- adenoma, thyroid gland   11
- cysts   119, 121
FSH levels, ovarian cysts   120

gastrinoma
- gastrointestinal tract   99, 100
- pancreas   99
gastrointestinal tract, endocrine tumors   99
gastrojejunostomy, pancreatic head tumor   98
germinal tumors, ovarian   113, 116
- and stroma tumors, mixed   113
glucagon, PINH   63
glucagonoma
- gastrointestinal tract   99, 100
- pancreas   99
glucose administration, nesidioblastosis   78
goitre/goiter (see also thyroid gland)   5–7, 11
- adenomatous changes   10
- diffuse toxic   34
- hyperfunctional diffuse   35
-- multinodular   35
- hyperthyroid   37
- juvenile   22
- multinodular toxic   34
- nodular   22, 38
- recurrence   36
gonadoblastoma, ovarian   113
gonadotropin, beta-human-chorionic (beta-
   HCG), ovarian tumors   116–118
granulosa cell tumor
- ovarian   113
-- stroma   115
Graves' disease   29, 38, 39, 51
- thyroid gland   6, 9, 16, 23

Hashimoto's
- disease   38
- thyroiditis   23, 39
HCG (human-chorionic gonadotropin)
- beta-HCG, ovarian tumors   116–118
- paraovarian cysts   122
von Hippel-Lindau disease, pheochromocytoma   106
homovannilic acid (HVA)

– neuroblastoma   125
– urinary, pheochromocytoma   108
hormone
– assay data, hyperthyroidism   34
– parathyroid   549
– substitution   28
– treatment, thyroid   32
– – substitution treatment, thyroid carcinoma
   44
HVA (homovannilic acid)
– neuroblastoma   125
– urinary, pheochromocytoma   107, 108
hypercalcemia
– familial hyperparathyroidism   52
– idiopathic infantile, hyperparathyroidism
   55, 56
– parathyroid hormone   50
– spontaneously primary hyperparathyroidism
   51
hyperinsulinism   77
– idiopathic neonatal   61
– nesidioblastosis   92, 93
– nesidioblastosis, total pancreatectomy
   92ff.
hyperparathyroidism   49, 53
– familial   52ff.
– persistent   54
– primary   50–52
– – infancy   55ff.
– – neonatal   55
– – spontaneous   51
– prolonged permanent   54
– recurrent   54
– secondary   50, 56
– solitary autosomal dominant   53
– tertiary   57
hypertension, pheochromocytoma   104, 105
hyperthyroid
– goitre   37
– struma, immunogenic   29, 30
– – treatment   29
– symptoms 33
hyperthyroidism   16, 17, 22, 28, 37, 38
– hormone assay data   34
– immune   17, 32
– immunogenic   29
– – treatment   29
– immunological assay data   35, 36
– juvenile   28ff.
– – subtotal resection   30
– – surgical treatment, after care   28ff.
– – surgical treatment, indications   28ff.
– late results of thyroid surgery   31ff.
– manifest   34–36
– – recurring   36

– nonimmunogenic   29
– postoperative   29
– radioiodine therapy   28
– recurrent   29, 30, 37
– subclinical   34–36
hypertonic dextrose, PINH   63
hypocalcemia
– secondary hyperparathyroidism   56
– spontaneously primary hyperparathyroidism
   51
hypocalciuric hypercalcemia
– familial (FHH)   53
– primary hyperparathyroidism   51
hypoglycemia   77
– idiopathic neonatal   60ff.
– insulin-induced, nesidioblastosis   78
– nesidioblastosis   93, 94
– PINH (persistent idiopathic neonatal
   hypoglycemia)   60ff.
hypokalemia, nesidioblastosis   85
hypoparathyroidism   33
– pharmacologic management   57
hypophysophatemia, parathyroid hormone
   50
hypothyroidism   22, 38

^{131}I   .
– supplement treatment, thyroid carcinoma
   43
– uptake   32
idiopathic neonatal
– hyperinsulinism   61
– hypoglycemia   61
immune
– globulins   38
– hyperthyroidism   17, 32
– thyroiditis   22
immunogenic
– hyperthyroid struma   29, 30
– hyperthyroidism, treatment   29
immunological
– assay data, hyperthyroidism   35, 36
– tests, thyroid carcinoma   46
immunopheotyping, neuroblastoma   125
insulin   65
– requirement   90
insulin-induced hypoglycemia, nesidioblastosis
   78
insulinoma
– gastrointestinal tract   99, 100
– pancreas   99
iodine
– deficiency   24, 25
– treatment, hyperthyroidism   28
iodized table salt prophylaxis   16, 23, 25

irradiation
- ^{60}Co iradiation, thyroid gland   24
- cobalt, thyroid carcinoma   43
islet cell/islets
- adenoma, nesidioblastosis   79
- adenomatosis, PINH   70
- dysplasia, PINH   61, 65, 66, 68
- formation, fetal, nesidioblastosis   92
- Langerhans, PINH   66, 90
- nuclear hypertrophy, PINH   68, 70
- proliferation, nesidioblastosis   93
- transplantation, insulin requirement   90
isolitary nodule   37

jejunum
- cholecystojejunostomy, pancreatic head
   tumor   98
- gastrojejunostomy, pancreatic head tumor
   98
- pancreaticojejunostomy, pancreatic head
   tumor   98
juvenile
- goiter   22
- hyperplasia, thyroid gland   22
- hypertyhroidism   28
- struma   16, 25

LAI (leucocyte adhesion inhibition), thyroid
   carcinoma   44
Langerhans, islets, PINH   66, 90
laryngeal nerve damage   54
leucocyte
- adhesion inhibition (LAI), thyroid
   carcinoma   42-44
- migration test, thyroid carcinoma   36,
   42, 43, 45
LH levels, ovarian cysts   120
LHRH stimulation, ovarian cysts   120
lingual thyroid (dystrophy of the thyroid
   gland)   5
lipoid cell tumor, ovarian   113
lobectomy   42
L-thyroxine 23-25, 29
Lugol's solution   32
lymph node
- matastasis   43
- regional   42
lymphocytic thyroiditis   38
- chronic   29

malign struma   19
malignant lymphoma, ovarian tumors   113
maternal hypoparathyroidism   55
MEA II (multiple endocrine adenomatosis
   syndrom II)

- hyperparathyroidism   54
- pheochromocytoma   105, 106
- syndrome, pheochromocytoma   106
MEN (multiple endocrine neoplasia)
- pancreatic head tumor   98
- type IIb   24
MEN II (multiple endocrine neoplasia II),
   pheochromocytoma   105
mesoblastic nephroma, hyperparathyroidism
   55
metabolig test, basal   32
metastasis
- thyroid carcinoma   42, 44
-- formation   42
- thyroid gland   6
migration index, thyroid gland   33
monoclonal antibodies, neuroblastoma   125
multinodular lesion   37
multiple endocrine neoplasia syndrome (see
   MEN)

N-myc
- messenger RNA, neuroblastoma   125
- oncogene, neuroblastoma   125
neck surgery, exploratory, spontaneous
   primary hyperparathyroidism   51
neonatal
- hyperparathyroidism   53
- hypoglycemia   61
- primary hyperparathyroidism   55
nesidioblastosis   76ff.
- adenoma   88
- clinical picture   77
- diagnosis   78
- focal adenomatosis   88
- incidence of recurrence   88
- multifocal proliferation   88
-- plus adenoma   88
- neonatal hypoglycemia   61
- pathohistological findings   88
- surgery   79-82, 84ff.
-- age at operation   81, 85
-- indications   76
-- conservative preoperative treatment   81
-- pancreatectomy, left-sided   86, 88, 89
-- pancreatectomy, near total   87, 94
-- pancreatectomy, subtotal   79-81,
   85-89
-- pancreatectomy, subtotal   92ff.
-- pancreatectomy, total   86-89, 92ff.
-- preoperative state   81
-- surgical procedure   85, 86
-- time for onset   81
- results   76
- treatment   76

neural ectodermal tumors, neuroblastoma
  125
neuroblastoma 124ff.
– biologic characteristics   125
– CCSG-staging   128
– complete surgical resection   128
– Evans staging system   128
– malignancies among infants   125
– nonresectable tumors   130
– pathologic diagnosis   125
– pediatric oncology group   128
– resectable tumors   129, 130
– surgery
– – "second-look" surgical procedures   127
– – supportive care   127
– – surgical management   127
– treatment   128
– tumor imaging   126, 127
neuroectodermal tumor, malignant ovarian
  115
neurotensinoma
– gastrointestinal tract   99, 100
– pancreas   99
nitroprusside, pheochromocytoma   108
nodular goitres   22, 38
nodule
– multinodular lesion   37
– solitary   37
norepinephrine, pheochromocytoma   104,
  107
normocalcemia after parathyroidectomy   53
nuclear
– DNA distribution   44
– hypertrophy, PINH   66

ophthalmological symptoms   33
ophthalmopathy   32, 34–36
– endocrine   29, 38
ovarian
– cystadenofibroma   115
– cystadenomas   114
– cysts   113, 114, 119
– dysgerminoma   117
– and germinal stroma tumors, mixed   113
– germinal tumors   116
– stroma, tumors   115
– teratomas   114, 116, 117
– – benign   114, 115
– tumor-like lesions   119
– tumor(s)
– – cysts   113
– – epithelial   115
– – histological diagnosis   115
– – pathohistological classifications   113
– – solid   114

– – surgical treatment   112ff.
– Yolk Sac tumors (endodermal sinus)   114
  115, 118
ovariectomy
– bilateral   116
– unilateral   116

pancreatectomy, nesidioblastosis   60ff., 71
– 85%   63, 64
– 95%   63–65
– left-sided   86, 88, 89
– near total   87, 94
– subtotal   79–81, 85–89
– total 86–89, 92ff.
pancreatic
– apudoma   97, 98
– carcinoid   97
– enzyme replacement   65
– head tumor   96ff.
– islet cells   77
– resection, methods   86
– tumors   98
– – endocrine   98
pancreaticojejunostomy, pancreatic head
  tumor   98
papillary thyroid carcinoma   18
paraovarian cysts   114, 121
parathyroid
– adenomas   51
– allotransplantation   57
– autotransplantation   54–57
– disease   49
– – diagnosis   50
– – pathophysiology   49
– disorders   49
– glands   49, 55
– hormone   49
– pathology   52
– surgery   48ff.
– syndromes   51
parathyroidectomy   50, 54
– normocalcemia   53
– total   55
PBI determination   32
pediatric oncology group staging, neuroblastoma   128
persistent idiopathic neonatal hypoglycemia
  (see PINH)   60ff.
phenoxybenzamine, pheochromocytoma   108
phentolamine, pheochromocytoma   108
pheochromacytoma   53, 103ff.
– diagnostic studies   106
– excision   109
– extra-adrenal   104
– symptoms   104

pheochromacytoma, treatment   108
phosphate concentration, parathyroid
  hormone   50
PINH (persistent idiopathic neonatal hypoglycemia)   60ff.
− histopathology   65
− immunohistochemistry   65
− medical management   63
− pathology   65
− surgery   62
− − surgical management   63
pituitary gland   52
postoperative
− hyperthyroidism   29
− hypoparathyroidism   30
− paralysis ot the recurrent nerve   30
− status, thyroid gland   5
postsplenectomy sepsis   88
pp-oma
− gastrointestinal tract   99, 100
− pancreas   99
preoperative thyroid metaboilsm, autonomous
  adenoma   30
prophylaxis
− iodized table salt prophylaxis   16, 23, 25
− struma endemic areas   25
− thyroid gland   24
propranolol, pheochromocytoma   108
pseudohypoparathyroidism   56
pTNM classification, thyroid carcinoma   42

radiation , ^{60}Co irradiation, thyroid gland   24
radioiodine treatment
− hyperthyroidism   28
− thyroid gland   24, 37, 38
radiotherapy, neuroblastoma   130
Recklinghausen disease, pheochromocytoma
  105, 106

salpingo-oophorectomy
− ovarian stroma   115
− ovarian tumors   122
salt, iodized table salt prophylaxis   16, 23, 25
sepsis, postsplenectomy   88
serous cystadenoma, ovarian   115
Sertoli-Leydig cell tumors, ovarian stroma
  115
Sipple syndrome   98
− pheochromocytoma   105
soft-tissue tumors, ovarian   113
solitary adenoma, nesidioblastosis   85
somatostatinoma
− gastrointestinal tract   99, 100
− pancreas   99
− pancreatic head tumor   97

sonographic imaging (see also ultrasound)
  1ff.
− thyroid gland   1, 12
staging of neuroblastoma   128, 129
struma
− cell tumor, ovarian   116
− colloides   23
− endemic areas, prophylaxis   25
− euthyroid   17
− hyperthyroid, immunogenic treatment   29
− immunogenic hyperthyroid   29, 30
− juvenile   16, 25
− maligna   19
− multifocal   30
− prevalence   16
− relapse   23
− retrosternal   22
− truma-endemic area   22, 24
strumectomy
− subtotal   17, 23
− total   17
substitution therapy, thyroid gland   17
supression tests   32
surgery
− neck, exploratory, spontaneous primary
  hyperparathyroidism   51
− nesidioblastosis   79
− parathyroid   48ff.
− PINH   62
− thyroid   37
− thyroid gland, benign and malignant
  diseases   21−27
surgical
− removal of thyroid tissue   28
surgical treatment juvenile hypertyhroidism
− after care   28ff.
− indications   28ff.
survival
− children, thyroid carcinoma   43
− rate, thyroid carcinoma   42
syndrome(s)
− blue diaper syndrome   55
− DeGeorge's syndrome   57
− MEA II syndrome, pheochromocytoma
  106
− Sipple syndrome   98
− − pheochromocytoma   105
− Verner-Morrison-syndrome, vipoma   100
− Whipple syndrome   98
− Zollinger-Ellison sydnrome   52
− − gastrinoma   100

T_3 uptake   32
T_3U
− test, thyroid carcinoma   46

– value, thyroid carcinoma   46
T₄
– concentration, thyroid carcinoma   46
– index (FT4I), thyroid carcinoma   46
T₄-RIA   32
– thyroid carcinoma   46
T-cell sensibilization, thyroid carcinoma   44
teratoma
– benign, ovarian   114, 115
– cystic, ovarian   116
– immature, ovarian   113
– malignant, ovarian   115, 116
– mature, ovarian   113
– ovarian   114, 116
testicular seminoma   117
tests
– basal metabolic test   32
– immunological tests, thyroid carcinoma   46
– leucocyte migration test   36, 42, 43, 45
– supression tests   32
– T₃U test, thyroid carcinoma   46
– TRH-loading tests   32
– TRH-TSH test   32
therapy (see treatment)   17
thyroglobulin, anti-human   33
thyroid
– autonomy   25
– carcinoma   5, 6, 11, 16, 18, 22, 37, 41ff.
– – anaplastic cancer   46
– – follicular   43, 44
– – immunlogical tests   46
– – late prognosis   41ff.
– – leucocyte adhesion   42, 43
– – leucocyte migration test   36, 42, 43, 45
– – medullary   43, 44, 46
– – metastasis formation   42
– – papillary   18, 43, 44
– – survival of the children   43
– – survival rate   42
– – tumour size   42
– – tumour-associated antigen   43
– enlargement   33
– function   34, 35, 42, 45
– gland
– ⁶⁰Co iradiation   24
– – abnormal imaging   5
– – abnormal of parenchymal echogenicity   6
– – abnormalities of size   5
– – adenoma   5, 6, 11, 23, 25
– – adenoma, autonomous   22, 29, 30,
  32–35, 37
– – adenoma, follicular   11
– – adenomatous changes, multiple   6
– – agenesis, lobe   5
– – agenesis, organ   5

– – anaplastic carcinoma   24
– – anatomy   2
– – aplasia, one lobe   5
– – benign diseases 23
– – bleeding   5
– – carcinoma/tumour   5, 6, 11, 16, 18, 24
– – cyst   5, 6
– – cyst, solitary small   10
– – dystrophy (lingual thyroid)   5
– – embryology   2
– – follicular carcinoma   24
– – goitre   5, 6, 11
– – Graves' disease   6, 9, 16, 23
– – hereditary influences   23
– – history, positive family   25
– – hyperthyroidism   16
– – hypoplasia of the organ   5
– – juvenile hyperplasia   22
– – medullary carcinoma (C-cell)   24, 53
– – metastasis   6
– – migration index   33
– – normal imaging   4
– – papillary carcinoma   24
– – pathological sonographic findings   5, 6
– – status   5
– – prophylaxis, recurrence   23, 25
– – radioiodine treatment   24, 37, 38
– – recurrence prophylaxis   24
– – right lobe, agenesis   7
– – sonographic imaging   1
– – sonography   1ff., 12
– – substitution therapy   17
– – surgical aspects   15–20
– – TSH-thyroid axis   22
– – tumour/carcinoma   5, 6, 11, 16, 18, 24
– hormone treatment   32
– hormones   38
– hyperfunction   32
– hypoplasia   6
– metabolism, preoperative, autonomous
  adenoma   30
– nodules   9, 19
– – multiple   9
– – solitary   9, 22
– parathyroid surgery   48ff.
– scan   32
– surgery   37
– – late results   31ff.
– tissue, surgical removal   28
thyroidectomy
– subtotal   42
– total   24, 42
thyroiditis   5, 6
– chronic lymphocitic   29
– focal   6, 8

thyroiditis, Hashimoto's   23
− immune   22
thyrostatic
− drugs   28, 29
− treatment   17
thyrotoxic crisis   29, 30, 32
thyrotropin   24
thyroxine
− L-thyroxine   23–25
− substitution   18
treatment
− antithyroid drug   32
− chemotherapy, ovarian tumors   117
− immunogenic
− − hyperthyroid struma   29
− − hyperthyroidism   29
− iodine, hyperthyroidism   28
− juvenile hypertyhroidism, surgical treatment   28ff.
− nesidoblastosis   76
− neuroblastoma   128
− thyroid
− − carcinoma, ^{131}I supplement   43
− − gland, radioiodine   24, 37, 38
− − hormone   32
− thyrostatic   17
TRH-loading tests   32
TRH-TSH test   32
TSH
− anti-TSH receptor antibody   33
− concentration, thyroid carcinoma   46
TSH-thyroid axis   22, 25
tuberous sclerosis, pheochromocytoma   106
tumor(s) (see carcinoma)
− ovarian stroma   115
− size, thyroid carcinoma   42
− thyroid gland   5, 6, 18, 19, 22, 24

tumour-associated antigen, thyroid carcinoma   43

ultrasound (see also sonographic imaging)   1ff.
− equipment   3
− examination technique   3
− thyroid gland   1ff.
urinary homovanillic acid (HVA), pheochromocytoma   108

vanillacetic acid, (VMA)   125
vanillylmandelic acid (VMA), neuroblastoma   125
Verner-Morrison-syndrome, vipoma   100
vipoma
− gastrointestinal tract   99, 100
− pancreas   99
vitamin D, parathyroid hormone   50
VMA (hydroxy-mandelic/vanillylmandelic acid)
− neuroblastoma   125
− pheochromocytoma   107
VMA:HVA ratio, neuroblastoma   125

Whipple
− procedure (duodenopancratectomy)   96
− syndrome   98

X-ray, thyroid carcinoma   43

Yolk Sac tumors, ovarian (endodermal sinus)   114, 115, 118

Zollinger-Ellison sydnrome   52
− gastrinoma   100

Progress in Pediatric Surgery

Co-founding Editor: P. P. Rickham

Editors: T. A. Angerpointner, M. W. L. Gauderer, W. Ch. Hecker, J. Prévot, L. Spitz, U. G. Stauffer, P. Wurnig

Volume 25

T. A. Angerpointner, University of Munich (Ed.)

Operative Technique in Neonates and Infants

1990. VIII, 141 pp. 77 figs., some in color. 34 tabs.
Hardcover DM 176,– ISBN 3-540-51057-5

This is the first volume of the **Progress in Pediatric Surgery** series devoted entirely to technical aspects. The chapters stem partly from papers presented at a symposium on the occasion of Prof. Hecker's 65th birthday and partly from invited contributions from authors who are expert in specialized technical procedures or have developed new surgical methods. The book thus gives an up-to-date overview of recent technical innovations in pediatric surgery.

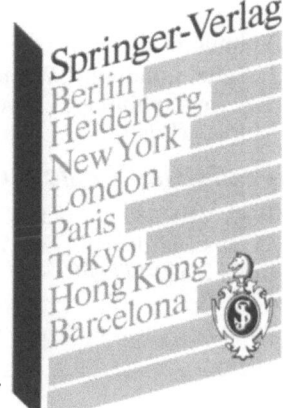

Springer-Verlag
Berlin
Heidelberg
New York
London
Paris
Tokyo
Hong Kong
Barcelona

Progress in Pediatric Surgery

Co-founding Editor: P. P. Rickham

Editors: T. A. Angerpointner, M. W. L. Gauderer, W. Ch. Hecker, J. Prévot, L. Spitz, U. G. Stauffer, P. Wurnig

Volume 24

J. Yokoyama, Keio University, Tokyo; T. A. Angerpointner, University of Munich (Eds.)

Constipation and Fecal Incontinence and Motility Disturbances of the Gut

1989. X, 235 pp. 113 figs. 62 tabs. Hardcover DM 198,–
ISBN 3-540-50813-9

Volume 23

L. Spitz, London; P. Wurnig, Vienna; T. A. Angerpointner, University of Munich (Eds.)

Surgery in Solitary Kidney and Corrections of Urinary Transport Disturbances

1989. VIII, 205 pp. 136 figs. 34 tabs. Hardcover DM 198,–
ISBN 3-540-50485-0

Volume 22

L. Spitz, London; P. Wurnig, Vienna; T. A. Angerpointner, University of Munich (Eds.)

Pediatric Surgical Oncology

1989. VIII, 180 pp. 78 figs. 44 tabs. Hardcover DM 178,–
ISBN 3-540-17769-8

Volume 21

P. Wurnig, Vienna (Ed.)

Trachea and Lung Surgery in Childhood

1987. X, 147 pp. 75 figs. Hardcover DM 136,–
ISBN 3-540-17232-7

Volume 20

P. P. Rickham, Zurich (Ed.)

Historical Aspects of Pediatric Surgery

1986. X, 285 pp. 119 figs. Hardcover DM 240,– ISBN 3-540-15960-6

Volume 19

P. Wurnig, Vienna (Ed.)

Long-gap Esophageal Atresia Prenatal Diagnosis of Congenital Malformations

1986. XII, 205 pp. 86 figs. Hardcover DM 180,– ISBN 3-540-15881-2

Prices are subject to change without notice.

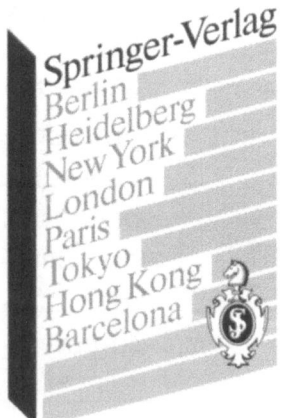

Springer-Verlag
Berlin
Heidelberg
New York
London
Paris
Tokyo
Hong Kong
Barcelona